Practical Horse Law

A Guide for Owners and Riders

Brenda Gilligan, *LLB*

Pritchard Englefield Solicitors

Blackwell
Science

© 2002 by Blackwell Science Ltd,
a Blackwell Publishing Company
Editorial Offices:
Osney Mead, Oxford OX2 0EL, UK
   Tel: +44 (0)1865 206206
Blackwell Science, Inc., 350 Main Street,
Malden, MA 02148-5018, USA
   Tel: +1 781 388 8250
Iowa State Press, a Blackwell Publishing
Company, 2121 State Avenue, Ames, Iowa
50014-8300, USA
   Tel: +1 515 292 0140
Blackwell Science Asia Pty, 54 University
Street, Carlton, Victoria 3053, Australia
   Tel: +61 (0)3 9347 0300
Blackwell Wissenschafts Verlag,
Kurfürstendamm 57, 10707 Berlin, Germany
   Tel: +49 (0)30 32 79 060

The right of the Author to be identified as
the Author of this Work has been asserted in
accordance with the Copyright, Designs and
Patents Act 1988.

First published 2002 by Blackwell Science
Ltd

Library of Congress
Cataloging-in-Publication Data
is available

ISBN 0-632-05673-8

A catalogue record for this title is available
from the British Library

Set in 10/12.5pt Palatino
by DP Photosetting, Aylesbury, Bucks
Printed and bound in Great Britain by
MPG Books Ltd, Bodmin, Cornwall

For further information on
Blackwell Science, visit our website:
www.blackwell-science.com

Contents

Preface

What is 'horse law' and why write a book about it? It is true to say that there is very little law which is directed solely at the horse world. The Riding Establishments Acts 1964 and 1970 are examples, but the law in general can increasingly be seen in an equine context. This book is written not as a technical legal handbook for students and lawyers, but as a practical guide to the use of the law in certain situations for horse owners and riders. It will try and tell you when the law may not be appropriate and give alternatives to formal legal procedures together with tips to avoid becoming involved in legal tangles in the first place.

For many years the rule of thumb in the horse world was *caveat emptor*. This is a Latin phrase which literally translates to 'let the buyer beware' but the phrase is not only used in the context of buying and selling horses and ponies or indeed other goods, which is where it originated. The principle can be extended to many situations. In the past, for instance, if you took a job as an instructor or a groom, very often there was little job security. If you lost your job you just shrugged and moved into the next job, putting it all down to experience. Your horse might be severely injured by being kicked by another in a field. The owner of the kicker might say sorry and that would be the end of it – that's horses for you, isn't it? Your riding lesson might come to an abrupt halt as you are determinedly bucked off, breaking your arm. Well, you suppose you should have hung on tighter shouldn't you? Certainly your instructor was yelling at you loudly enough to do so!

But things have changed. Some think this is for the worse. Yes, horses are unpredictable; they do change character in different environments and they cannot be relied on. They are not dead lumps of metal like cars and they do have minds of their own. It is also accepted that riding is a risk sport and that we all fall off from time to time, even from the quietest horse, and it may well be a pure accident and no-one's fault.

But look at it the other way. You are a genuine buyer and willing to pay a fair price for the right horse. You make your requirements very clear to the seller of the horse – perhaps you are a novice rider and need a steady horse on which to gain confidence. You might tell them that you are looking to buy a talented jumper to compete on or a horse that can do medium level dressage. You are being as honest as you can and you are relying on the seller to be equally fair with you. Why then should you have no come-back when, having relied on a seller's assurances and handed over your precious saved money, you get the horse home to discover it really isn't what it was sold as and the seller must have known that? Why should you as the 'innocent party' have to suffer the loss and the problem of getting rid of a confirmed rearer? Equally, there has to be protection for the sellers from buyers who merely change their mind about having a horse after a few weeks and invent all sorts of reasons as to why the horse should be taken back.

It is the same with jobs. Employees need some sort of job security and employers do need to have a means of getting rid of unsuitable employees. If you are injured in an accident and it is clearly someone else's fault, then you need a remedy. Your injuries may be very serious causing you to lose earnings or even to require specialist long-term care, equipment and housing, all of which must be paid for.

Horse law doesn't just cover arguments and accident claims. You may want to set up a horse business such as a riding school, or you may want to run a show and need some guidance about to how to go about it and what is required. You might want to put your horse out on loan and need an agreement drawn up, or you might want to know whether you can put up a stable in your garden without planning permission. The law touches and concerns, to a greater or lesser degree, all aspects of the horse world.

Why are we turning to law more these days? Interest in horses is growing, and riding and owning horses is becoming more and more popular. There are therefore more people who need information and more people to make complaints.

There is also much more emphasis these days on our rights. As consumers, customers, employees, business people, etc., we have a better knowledge of what we are, or should be, entitled to, and others know what they have a right to expect from us. We are much more safety conscious and this has been underlined in the early 2000s by the focus on minimising the risks and improving safety in the sport following the untimely deaths of a number of event riders in a very short time. Some say that the fear of litigation is taking all the challenge and fun out of what is after all a risk sport, but the trick is to balance the removal of unnecessary and disproportionate risks with the need to retain a real challenge for appropriately experienced horses and riders. It can be done and it often only takes a few adjustments to make things safer. We should also remember that with rights come responsibilities. Yes, you have a right to ride your horse on the road, but this does not mean that you can ride a maniac over which you have little control in busy traffic and expect everyone else to keep out of your way. You have a responsibility to other road users to take care for their safety as well. You may well have a right to enter any standard of competition you like, even if your horse is not fit or not quite up to it. But who is going to look after you when you fall and suffer severe permanent injuries? Don't you have a responsibility towards your family to ride at a sensible level?

In law you don't have to eliminate every risk, you just have to take reasonable care, which is common sense.

Another factor in the increase in litigation could be the growth of insurance. Previously, it was often not worth trying to pursue a case (say, an accident claim) because even if you won, there would be no money to pay your damages, and it would be a pointless victory. More and more people these days are becoming insured and therefore there is more chance that people can afford to take on or defend a case and either pay compensation if unsuccessful or be awarded damages if they prove their claim, be it accident or otherwise.

The legal profession used to be seen as remote and inaccessible and 'taking legal advice' or 'seeing your solicitor' was a very serious and costly business. Many people were deterred from even seeking further information or investigating whether a claim might be viable. The legal profession itself has changed radically. There are now many solicitors willing to give free initial advice, and fees have become more competitive and affordable. There are advice centres, help lines, legal problem pages in magazines and generally more information around. Solicitors are now also willing to work on a 'no win, no fee' basis, for which the correct name is a Conditional Fee Agreement – a scheme designed to give access to legal advice and the justice system for a much wider range of people.

It is also true that we are perhaps now more willing to complain and seek redress for what we see as a wrong. Complaining can be effective where there is a genuine problem which can be remedied, but beware of complaining just because something has not turned out as you hoped. On the other hand, it may be helpful to a company for customers to complain. If a company receives a number of the same sort of complaint, it may wish to investigate and perhaps alter production methods. For example, horse owners might notice horses having a bad reaction to a feed supplement, or several owners might report a rug strap breaking under similar conditions.

It is not the intention of this book to encourage people to go to their solicitor threatening days in court at the slightest suspicion of wrong-doing. Rather, it is hoped that it will help you to avoid problems in the first place, while explaining the laws that are there to assist you when necessary. Most problems can usually be resolved or compromised over and this will reduce both the costs and the time taken to settle matters. There will, however, undoubtedly be cases where there is no alternative to legal proceedings and in those circumstances it is best to get yourself a good lawyer.

Acknowledgements

Acknowledgements and grateful thanks are due to the following for assistance with this book: The British Horse Society for a wealth of background information and kind permission to use and reproduce material produced and published by the society. Professor Barry Peachey and The Equine Lawyers Association for much background information, particularly case law, and kind permission to use and quote from material produced and published by the ELA particularly the journal of the association 'Horse Law – The Equine Law and Litigation Reports'. Butterworths Publishers for background information from Halsbury's Laws and Halsbury's Statutes. The Medical Equestrian Association for information on equestrian safety issues, injuries and treatment. The Association of British Riding Schools for discussion and information about their work. British Equestrian Insurance Brokers for information on insurance policies. David Mountford from the International League of Protection for Horses for his time in explaining the work of the ILPH. The Veterinary Defence Union for explaining the work of the VDU. The British Equine Veterinary Association for background information on vetting procedures with reference to the BEVA publication 'The Pre-Purchase Examination'. Mary Lou Lees and Bev Rippon of the British Equine Dental Technicians Association for information on the association and equine dental procedures generally. Peter Green, veterinary surgeon of Fellowes Farm Equine Clinic, Huntingdon, for the extended loan of his book and information on vetting procedures. Antony and Andrew from Peaceful Pets for enlightenment on the mysteries of equine cremation and disposal. Brian Bates and the National Trailer and Towing Association for enthusiastic information on trailers and towing. The author's secretaries Linda and Rachel for typing the words, Ian Griffiths for his IT assistance and colleagues at Pritchard Englefield for their help and support. The 'focus group' at the author's stable yard for their opinions. Mark and Stephanie for their ability to turn a computer on and off without losing everything. Carlad, Drummer and Mouse, for being horses.

Disclaimer

This book has been written for the lay horse owner and rider as a broad general guide to the law and legal situations where advice may be needed. It is not, nor does it pretend to be, the definitive text on the law in every given situation – each case is individual and requires specific advice on its own facts at the time. The law and its interpretation changes constantly and rapidly. What might be the case today may not be tomorrow.

It is strongly recommended that readers consult a specialist solicitor or take other appropriate independent advice before drafting or drawing up any document or letter; committing themselves to any action or omission; where they find themselves wondering what their rights might be in a situation; or indeed if they have any rights at all. Advice should be sought as soon as possible.

Neither the author, any partner or member or staff of Pritchard Englefield nor the publishers can or will be liable to anyone who suffers any adverse consequence, loss, damage or injury, in any form whatsoever, as a result of any action taken or omitted as a result of directly or indirectly relying on the contents of this book whether independent advice has been sought or not.

The opinions expressed are the author's own and are not necessarily those of Pritchard Englefield or other members of the legal profession or other advisors.

Chapter 1
Regulation of Riding Establishments

Many people start their riding career by having lessons at a riding school. If you look at old pony books, they are full of stories of people, including children, starting up their own riding schools to help raise money to keep their ponies who would otherwise have to be sold, or to make use of some unused stables around the farm where they happen to live. These days, thankfully, riding schools are more regulated and need to be licensed to operate as a school. The licence will only be granted when certain conditions have been fulfilled.

Livery yards do not need licences to operate, although if they do partly carry out the function of a riding school they will need to have a licence. Yards can seek approval from the British Horse Society, which produces an information pack with guidance on how to gain approval. It is neither mandatory to apply nor for the British Horse Society to grant. You can run a livery yard without any sort of licence or approval from the BHS, but to get BHS approval you will need to reach certain minimum standards with regard to running the yard, care of the animals, etc., and there is also a code of conduct which must be adhered to, a copy of which can be obtained from the BHS. The BHS will inspect regularly. Riding schools need a local authority licence and can apply for BHS or Association of British Riding Schools (ABRS) approval. Livery yards do not need the local authority licence, but can apply for BHS approval as a mark of respectability, if you like.

Livery yards will be covered in Chapter 8.

There are several good reasons for having lessons at a proper riding school. One of the main ones is that as well as having to conform to certain standards, licensed stables are required to be insured against any liabilities for injury to their paying customers caused by the stables' negligence. Having said that, it is not the intention of the writer to give the impression that all lessons will end in disaster. The vast majority of riding lessons pass entirely without incident, but even in the best-run schools there will be accidents for which compensation may be justified.

Compensation awards in this country are generally regarded as not being high for the injury. As an example there is the case of *Crowe* v. *Shana*

Riding School and Buckinghamshire Health Authority (2000) (*Horse Law*, Vol. 5, Iss. 3). This case was a little unusual as it concerned both personal injury and clinical negligence. The claimant, Ms Crowe, broke her back falling from a horse at the riding school and she was awarded damages because it was found that the horse was not suitable for her to learn to ride. Unfortunately, when Ms Crowe was taken to hospital, her treatment there was not as good as it should have been and eventually the hospital was also found to be negligent. The damages, which amounted to £700,000 were apportioned to be paid partially by the riding school and partially by the hospital. £700,000 may seem a lot of money, but in personal injury cases, damages running into millions are not unusual and you may find it surprising that you will now routinely be advised to take out third party liability cover up to £10 million. Riding schools are required to have third party insurance under the terms of the licence granted by the local authority under the Riding Establishments Acts. Horse owners/riders and even those who just ride, even if they don't own a horse but ride other people's horses, should have at least third party liability insurance. If you are a member of a recognised body, e.g. the British Horse Society, membership will very often include insurance so the joining fee is worthwhile.

Licensing a riding school

Acts governing riding schools are the Riding Establishments Acts 1964 and 1970. They are usually spoken of together, although the 1964 Act is the principal or main Act. The 1970 Act merely makes provision for a provisional licence to be granted for a short time. The 1964 Act provides that no-one can keep a riding establishment unless they hold a licence from the local authority, which will probably be your local county council. If you apply for a licence, you should first have acquired your premises and checked that all is in order with regard to planning permissions, rates, staffing, issues, etc. The Acts apply to Scotland as well as England and Wales, but not Northern Ireland.

A riding school is described in section 6(1) of the Act as 'the carrying on of a business of keeping horses for either or both of the following purposes . . . being let out for hire or riding or . . . being used in providing, in return for payment, instruction in riding'. The Acts do not apply to riding schools under the management of the Secretary of State for Defence (i.e. army horses) nor to the police, or to horses kept by the Zoological Society of London, or the horses kept by universities training veterinary students. Your establishment can therefore be called a riding school if you only let out horses for hacking or if you provide instruction. If the purpose of your yard is to provide facilities for horses to be kept, even if the owners of those horses then have lessons on them, it would not be classified as a riding school. An instructor giving you lessons on your own horse would not be classified as a riding school.

Unless you specify otherwise, the riding school will be taken to be situated at the place where the horses used for the business are kept.

If you are in any doubt as to whether or not your establishment qualifies as a riding school then you should contact your local authority immediately to clarify the position as it is a criminal offence to run a riding school without a licence. There is a fee for the licence, which may differ with each local authority and may for instance depend on the number of horses you have on the premises; if the licence is granted it will be for the premises specified in the licence. There may be some specific conditions attached to it; for instance, there may be a limit on the number of horses you can have. The licence remains in force for one calendar year, either from the day it is granted or at the beginning of the next following year according to the applicant's requirements, and then it expires. Under the Riding Establishments Act 1970, a provisional licence for three months can be granted and this can be extended for a further three months, but you cannot have a provisional licence for more than six months in any period of one year.

You will not be granted a licence if:

(1) You are under 18.
(2) You are disqualified from keeping a riding establishment having committed an offence under the Act.
(3) You are disqualified from keeping a pet shop.
(4) You are disqualified from keeping animals under the Protection of Animals Act 1954 or from boarding animals under the Animal Boarding Establishments Act 1963.

The local authority can withhold a licence at their discretion. However, if they did so without giving a proper explanation as to why, you might be able to challenge the decision under the Riding Establishment Act through the magistrates' court or even by way of judicial review. A judicial review is a legal procedure whereby a court looks at decisions made by public bodies to see if they are 'reasonable decisions reasonably made'. The court would not be concerned with whether the decision was right, just whether it had been reached on reasonable arguments and principles. Under the Act, there is a right of appeal to a Magistrates' Court and if you need to do this you will almost certainly need the assistance of a solicitor.

The local authority have to consider specific matters when considering whether to grant a licence and these are set out in section 1(4) of the Act, broadly as set out below. In granting a licence they will only be looking at the riding school and the riding school horses, so if you have a mixed livery/riding school yard they will not necessarily look at the liveries or indeed your own horses when considering whether to grant a licence. It would be prudent, however, to ensure that the same standards are adhered to whether the horses are riding school horses or not.

Points considered by the local authority

The local authority will consider whether the person making the application appears to be a suitable person to run a riding school. You can demonstrate your suitability either by experience or by having approved qualifications 'in the management of horses'. You can have an 'approved certificate', defined as a British Horse Society Assistant Instructor, Instructor or Fellowship Certificate, Fellowship of the Institute of the Horse or any other certificate allowed by law.

British Equestrian Tourism have three different levels of qualification. These are Assistant Ride Leader, Ride Leader and Holiday Riding Centre Manager. The Assistant is trained to accompany short hacks with up to six riders, or to assist a Ride Leader on larger group hacks or over a longer distance. The Ride Leader can take sole charge of hacks, whether novices or experienced riders. Both should have a knowledge of safety and be able to help in the running of a yard, with the Ride Leader able to deputise in running the yard completely if necessary. Both these qualifications would be more suited to trekking or leisure riding centres. The level of Holiday Riding Centre Manager will be someone who is trained to run a centre in business terms, i.e. financially, and can advise on the operation of such centres. Again, this may be more suited to the tourism and leisure side of equestrian business.

You can also be given a licence if you can show that you employ someone with these qualifications or relevant experience to manage the school.

The overriding factor in the local authority's decision on whether to grant a licence will be the condition and health of the horses and their suitability as riding school horses. This does not necessarily mean that they all have to be 'plods'; clearly a specialised dressage school would want well-schooled horses capable of doing dressage and a specialised showjumping yard would want horses capable of showjumping, which may not necessarily be suitable for beginners or novices. The average riding school probably has a variety of types, but the local authority will be looking at whether the horse is suitable for the purpose for which it is kept.

The local authority will also consider the following factors:

(1) Horses' feet must be looked after, properly shod and trimmed.
(2) Stabling, new or converted, must be suitable in all respects – size, ventilation, lighting, etc.
(3) Horses kept at grass should have 'adequate pasture... shelter and water... with supplementary feed as necessary'.
(4) Horses must have adequate provision of food, water and bedding and must be exercised, groomed, rested and supervised regularly.
(5) There must be first-aid equipment on the premises and precautions in place to prevent the spread of infectious or contagious diseases.
(6) There must be adequate fire prevention measures and a rescue plan for horses in the event of fire. The name, address and telephone number of the licence holder or some other responsible person must be prominently displayed together with instructions as to what to do in the event of fire.
(7) There must be adequate accommodation and storage facilities for feed, equipment, bedding and saddlery.

The key words in all this are somewhat subjective – 'adequate', 'regularly' 'properly'. There is no specific definition of what is adequate, regular or proper, but if you look at it the other way round, inadequate provision would be fairly obvious – ten horses on an acre of grass, a stable too small for a horse to turn round or lie down in. It is always recommended that horses are checked at least twice a day, but regular supervision could be more if necessary, for instance for a sick horse.

You will probably be doing things 'properly' if you are using suitably qualified people for the purpose, a farrier for instance (we are presuming that the farrier is doing his job correctly), or if you are following some sort of guidelines, British Horse Society or ABRS recommendations for instance. If you are not doing this, you won't necessarily be doing things improperly. The inspectors will not be always looking for the 'gold' standard. Not everyone can afford purpose-built stables with infra-red lights, but neither are they essential for a horse's well-being.

Even if you don't comply with all of these points on the first application, you could try again as the local authority could give you a licence with certain conditions to ensure that the objects are met, most likely within a certain time.

Essential conditions

There are certain conditions that every licence requires and these *cannot* be excluded or appealed. These are:

(1) If a local authority inspector inspects the premises and finds a horse needing veterinary attention, then before that horse is allowed to return to work the licence holder must produce a veterinary certificate to show that the horse is fit for work.

(2) Unless the holder of the licence is satisfied that a person hiring a horse is competent to ride the horse without supervision, no horse must be let out for hire or used for providing instruction in riding without supervision by a responsible person over 16 years of age. In all cases, no-one under 16 shall be left in charge of the riding school. (This is an important point when we consider accidents and safety in Chapter 14. It is suggested that no-one should be allowed to ride unsupervised.)

(3) The licence holder must have a current insurance policy insuring him or her against liability for any injury sustained by those who hire a horse from him or her for riding and those who use the horse in the course of receiving from him or her, in return for payment, instruction in riding where the injury arises out of that hire or instruction.

(4) The licence holder must keep a register of horses aged three and under which are usually kept on the premises in his possession and the register must be available for inspection.

Offences

You can be imprisoned, fined or disqualified from keeping horses for offences under the Riding Establishment Act. You must not:

- Use a horse whose condition means it would suffer when ridden.
- Use a horse under the age of three, or a horse heavily in foal or within three months of foaling.
- Supply riding equipment, for a horse let out on hire by you, which has a defect that could be seen on inspection and which is likely to cause suffering to the horse or accident to the rider.
- Fail to treat sick or injured horses.
- Knowingly let someone who is disqualified from running a riding establishment have control of or management of the riding school. 'Knowingly' can mean suspecting but failing to make proper enquiries which if made would lead you to find out that a person was disqualified. Always be very careful to take up references and incorporate a probationary period into any employment contract. You should also make it an offence punishable by summary dismissal, i.e. instant dismissal, if you find out someone has been disqualified, or has done something which would disqualify them.

- Conceal or cause to be concealed with the intent to avoid inspection any horse maintained by the riding establishment. This would mean, for instance, trying to hide a horse that was in poor condition during an inspection.

If information given for the purpose of obtaining a licence is false, it can be an offence under the Act.

Under section 5 of the Act, any legal proceedings against the proposed licence holder or the licence holder would be brought by the local authority, but they can only do that after they have considered a report from a vet which indicates that an offence has been committed. It is beyond the scope of this chapter to set out the many arguments and defences that can occur, and if you are facing prosecution by the local authority you should seek legal advice immediately.

Veterinary report

The local authority cannot make a final decision in the granting of a riding school licence unless they have received a considered report by a veterinary surgeon or practitioner following an inspection of the premises carried out within a period of 12 months before the application is made. The veterinary report will contain particulars as to whether the premises are suitable for a riding establishment, and will describe the condition of the premises and any horses found there.

Inspections

Once granted a licence, riding schools can expect to be inspected during the period of a licence, or on application for a new licence, either at very short notice or without any notice at all. However, the frequency and nature of the checks will vary depending on the availability and qualifications of the staff in each local authority. For inspections, you may get Environmental Health and Health and Safety Officers attending together with a vet. The vet may check each horse – eyes, heart, wind, etc. – check for any injuries, specifying those caused by any ill-fitting tack, and will look at the state of the horse's feet. The horse may be walked out and trotted up. Some vets will check the tack while others will not, but it is of course prudent to check that all tack is of a good make, in good condition and comfortable for each horse.

Each horse will have its own records including a personal description, which is kept by the county council/local authority and the vet. This is to try to avoid horses being substituted. The feed and hay will be checked, as will the storage facilities. Fencing, pasture, electrics and general safety in the yard and machinery will be looked at. You will need to have available for inspection your register of horses aged three and under and your accident report book. Very often, the qualifications of the staff are not checked, just those of the licence holder. It is probably a safeguard for you as the licence holder, however, if you do have properly qualified and experienced staff.

You will be told there and then whether you have passed the inspection and if not, you may be given a list of failures and a period in which to rectify them. Alternatively your licence may be withdrawn and you will have to apply for another one.

Endorsement by other organisations

Although the licence to run a riding school is mandatory, i.e. you must have it, there are other endorsements you may want to achieve, such as the British Horse Society or Association of British Riding Schools registrations. The British Horse Society can check your school without warning at any time, but will inspect at least annually and can remove you from their register if you don't come up to standard. If you are advertising yourself as giving tuition at a high standard, say specialist dressage or showjumping, then the British Horse Society will want to see evidence that this can be achieved, by watching lessons and checking that the horses are of a suitable grade for such lessons. You will need a British Horse Society qualified instructor doing the teaching. The ABRS offer a series of graded tests for pupils and teachers. They will also inspect and have a committee to deal with and rule on complaints made against members. The advantage of these endorsements lies in attracting clients and possibly being able to obtain special discounts on insurance policies.

Employing staff

If you run your riding school or livery yard as a business, or you have a business within it, such as a tack shop or tea shop, you may want to employ staff. Even if you just keep your horses at home on a non-profit making basis you may want someone to help out. If this is the case then you will need to comply with various employment laws and regulations. Some employment legislation only applies to businesses with a certain number of staff, but it is worth checking your legal position before taking on any staff. For instance, if you already employ a number of staff but feel you need more, consider whether taking on that extra one or two workers is going to take you into the area where many more laws apply. Can you afford the time and expense of complying with many more rules and regulations, or can you rearrange your current staff to work more effectively?

Employment law is probably one of the most challenging areas of law today, not only in its breadth and complexity but because of the rapidity of the changes. It is probably the area of law which tries hardest to keep up with current social practices and the reality of life, and is greatly affected by European law. It is a very complicated area of law and it is easy to fall behind on what is current owing to the number and pace of changes. It is also an area of law where time limits are extremely important. As an employee, if you do not comply with time limits for doing various things then you may lose any right you have to make claims for such things as unfair dismissal or discrimination claims. Legal Services Commission Funding (formerly Legal Aid) is not available for tribunal hearings, but it is common to find a solicitor who will take on your case on the basis that legal fees can be paid from any compensation you receive. Do remember that as an employer you have a duty of care towards your employees to keep them safe and offer a safe working environment, complying with the Health and Safety Regulations where appropriate, and you may also be liable for the actions of your employees if they are negligent and their actions result in injury or damage to others.

Choosing staff

As a brief overview, when taking on staff you will have to be prepared to comply with anti-discrimination laws and not reject someone for a job purely on the basis of whatever gender, colour or religion they are. A few years ago the King's Troop Royal Horse Artillery advertised for new recruits. They had not anticipated that women would apply and refused them access to the jobs. A Miss Emily Avis applied and was rejected. She duly complained on discriminatory grounds and her complaint was upheld. She was awarded £4500 in compensation.

However, think carefully if you are applying for a job where you will be the only male or the only female. Despite the law, circumstances and atmosphere can combine, while remaining within the law, to make things difficult for you, although the law does not allow 'harassment'. On the other hand, there always has to be a first and if you are sure that a certain job is what you want to do and you can cope with it, then go for it and stick with it. If you are successful, you will make it easier for those who come after you. Employment is changing all the time and what was not acceptable five years ago can be commonplace now.

You will not necessarily be able to reject someone purely because they are disabled. If you have an existing employee who becomes disabled you may be obliged under the Disability Discrimination Act 1995 to make reasonable changes to the working environment to allow that worker to resume their employment, or to offer suitable alternative work if available. The Disability Discrimination Act is a relatively recent Act and as yet there is not much case law on it to know how it is going to work, but it has the potential to be an interesting piece of legislation. How far, for instance, does an employer have to go in modifying or adapting surroundings to enable someone to continue work? In an office environment it may be a simple matter of putting in ramps and widening doorways to allow someone in a wheelchair to move around freely, but it may not be so easy to adapt an equine environment. If you are an employee who is injured and becomes disabled, are you going to be required to actively enforce the Disability Discrimination Act in order to enable yourself to go back to work, rather than claiming that you cannot go back to work because of your injuries and making a claim for benefits, or loss of earnings if you have a potential accident claim? It will be necessary to see what sort of cases are brought and what are the outcomes.

As an employer, you must have an Equal Opportunities Policy. The Equal Opportunities Commission, the Commission for Racial Equality and the Department for Work and Pensions under the Disability Discrimination Act produce Codes of Practice which are helpful.

Contracts of employment

When you take on someone as an employee, you are in most cases obliged to give them written particulars of employment. Certain terms will be implied in their employment which will apply whether they are written down or not. In any standard contract of employment, you will want for instance:

- Employer and employee's name and address.
- Where the employee's place of work is. Will the employee be expected to work at different places? If so, where and when?
- Date when job starts / date of 'continuous employment' if, for instance, the business has been sold but to all intents and purposes everything remains the same, including the employees.
- Description of job and employee's job title, if any, duties, hours of work, holidays, sickness leave, amount of wages, overtime entitlement, bonuses, pensions.
- Will the employee be allowed to do any other work – e.g. undertake private teaching? Can they use their employer's facilities for this?
- Is any accommodation, use of transport or own horse livery provided? If so, on what terms?

- Length of contract if not a permanent job.
- Notice periods.
- Any restrictive covenants – are you going to try to limit for whom the employee can work if they leave, or the geographical area in which they can work? You can usually only restrict these for a time, not for ever. The restrictions must be reasonable. What is deemed reasonable will differ in each individual case, but broadly speaking, any restrictions will be limited to what is reasonable to protect a business.
- Disciplinary procedures when the employer is unhappy with the employee's work, and grievance procedures where the employee has a complaint.

The above should not be taken as definitive or as the only terms that should be in a contract. The wording and content can be crucial if there is a dispute. A solicitor will draft a suitable basic contract to suit your business, and this can then be modified for each employee if necessary. Try to get advice from a solicitor who specialises in employment law.

Dismissal of staff

You will need to be aware of when you can and can't dismiss someone. Unfair dismissal is when somebody is literally dismissed unfairly. There are circumstances in which you can dismiss people quite legitimately and there are even circumstances where you can dismiss them summarily for a gross breach of conduct such as theft or, in an equine context, cruelty to the horses in their care. The circumstances in which summary dismissal is justified should be clearly set out in the contract of employment or policy document.

Wrongful dismissal is where somebody is dismissed in breach of their contract. The most common situation is failing to give the correct notice. An unfair dismissal hearing will be heard before an employment tribunal whereas a wrongful dismissal claim can be heard in a normal civil court as it is technically a breach of contract claim. An employment tribunal can award compensation of up to £25,000 for a wrongful dismissal claim.

Compensation can be awarded in both cases. In unfair dismissal claims there are two types of award – 'basic' and 'compensatory'. Up to £51,700 can be awarded as a compensatory claim, which is, as its name suggests, compensation for the financial losses consequent on being unfairly dismissed. The basic award is a figure dependent on the employee's pay, age and length of service. The tribunal can also offer jobs back, but realistically this is usually impractical. Wrongful dismissal claims are breach of contract claims and compensation will depend on what the employee could have expected under the contract had it been continued.

Insurance is available for the possibility of such claims being made against you as an employer.

Redundancy

Redundancy is another area to consider. In general terms, redundancy occurs when a job disappears, or when the need for a specific individual to do a certain job ceases. It is not just when you as the employer decide you do not want someone to do a specific job any more. An employee can claim unfair dismissal for having been made redundant incorrectly. Employees can, however, choose to be made redundant voluntarily. If you think you need, or want, to make staff redundant, do take legal advice as to whether or not it is legal to do so.

Health and safety

As mentioned previously, you will have to be sure that you comply with the Health and Safety at Work Act 1974. There is a general duty of employers to their employees to ensure, so far as is reasonably practicable, the health, safety and welfare at work of all the employees. In particular, as far as reasonably practicable the employer must:

- Provide and maintain plant and systems of work that are safe and without risks to health.
- Ensure that the use, handling, storage and transport of articles and substances are safe and do not present a risk to employees.
- Provide training, instruction, information and supervision to ensure health and safety at work. There must be provision and maintenance of 'any place under the employer's control' and the means of access and exit from it must be safe and without risk to health. Generally speaking, there must be provision of a working environment for employees that is safe, without risks to health, and adequate with regard to facilities and arrangements for their welfare at work.
- The employer must prepare and revise a written statement of the general policy with respect to health and safety and this must be brought to the notice of all employees. The employer has a similar duty to those not in their employment but who may be affected by anything on their premises and self-employed people have the same duty to themselves. Certain accidents and 'dangerous occurrences' at work, whether to an employee or someone at the place of work but not employed there must be reported by law to the Health and Safety Executive under the Reporting of Injuries, Diseases and Dangerous Occurrences Regulations 1995 (RIDDOR). Details of RIDDOR's useful

website on how to do this are given under Health and Safety Executive in 'Useful Addresses' at the back of this book.

This of course is not the entirety of the Health and Safety at Work regulations but just brings the basic requirements to the attention of employers. Do take specific advice on your obligations on health and safety.

The minimum wage

There have been some recent changes in employment law which may well have more specific impact on the horse world than the general employment law.

It is no secret that pay in the equine world has not always been of the highest and it has been common to offer training or work in exchange for accommodation and board, perhaps livery for your horse and literally pocket money. However, since 1 April 1999 the National Minimum Wage Regulations 1999 brought in by the National Minimum Wage Act 1998 have been enforced. You cannot contract out of the provisions of these regulations and they apply to 'workers' and not simply employees. Workers are, generally speaking, either an individual working under a contract of employment or any other contract for work. The regulations apply to:

- *Time work* – This is work paid for depending on the time a worker works and includes time when he or she is required to be available at or near the place of work and time spent travelling for the purpose of the duties. This could for instance include stud workers who are required to be on hand in case of problems and may have to travel to and from work for mares foaling at odd hours.
- *Salaried hours work* – This is where the worker has a certain number of basic hours which they are obliged to work. They may well work more hours but not necessarily get paid for these. This would include time required to be at or near the place of work and time spent travelling. Salaried workers can be paid for the extra hours they work at the national minimum wage rate, but only if the hourly rate during the course of the year, taking into account all the hours of work, would fall below the national minimum wage if you didn't pay for the extra hours.
- *Output work* – This is strictly speaking working on commission – where you get paid, for instance, by the number of pieces of clothing that you produce if you are a machinist, or the number of double glazing units you sell if you are a double glazing salesman.

- *Unmeasured work* – This is where the work has no specified hours but the worker is required to work when needed. Time spent travelling to and from work is not counted. Under this heading, the worker and the employer can enter into an agreement setting out the average daily number of hours the worker is likely to spend working and this would be the basis for calculating the minimum hourly rate.

Benefits and accommodation

One other point of interest to the horse world will be that benefits in kind are disregarded when calculating the minimum wage, but there is an allowance for living accommodation, at the time of writing up to a maximum of £3.25 per day or £27.75 per week, even if the 'commercial value' of this benefit would actually be more. (These figures are as at October 2001 and are likely to be subject to change from time to time.) Therefore, even if you give your staff rent-free accommodation say to the market value of £80 per week, you would only be allowed to take into account £27.75 towards what you should pay them under the minimum wage regulations. Benefits such as livery for a student's horse would be completely ignored so you would have to pay the minimum wage plus the cost of livery if you were thinking of offering this sort of arrangement. This could mean that it becomes unattractive for employers to offer this sort of package, with the result that many students will not be able to bring their horses with them on taking up employment.

If you have a 'worker', again using the example of say a stud groom, who is required to be 'at or near his place of work other than his home' for the purposes of doing work, then they may need to be paid the national minimum wage even if they are not actively doing anything; e.g. they are just on call in case a mare foals. You will note that the regulations say that they have to be at or near their place of work, but not at home for this to apply. You might run into a problem where accommodation is provided near the place of work, as many stables do offer their staff. From an employer's point of view, if the accommodation provided is actually the worker's home then time spent there may not be considered working time and will not have to be paid for. From the employee's point of view, however, this may be unsatisfactory because they may feel that even though they are 'at home' they are really 'on duty' and liable to be called in at any time if a problem arises, but they will not be paid for this time. Because the regulations are fairly new there are few cases and no doubt this will be clarified. Take specialist advice if you can before entering into this sort of arrangement, or if this is not possible, then take advice on how the regulations might affect you and whether there are any steps you should be taking as an employer or employee.

Minimum wage rates

The minimum wage rates change from time to time. Rather than set them out here where they may become out of date, it is best to check the current ones with the Department of Trade and Industry or the citizens' advice bureau when you are considering taking on staff. The DTI can be contacted on 0845 6000 678 or via their website at www.dti.gov.uk/er/nmw. There is also a specific website for minimum wage rate queries at www.tiger.gov.uk. (Tiger stands for 'Tailored Interactive Guidance on Employment Rates'). As of 1 October 2001 the rates are £4.10 per hour for workers aged 22 or above and £3.50 per hour for those aged 18 to 21. An exception to this are trainees in the first twelve months of a government training scheme. There are different rates for those who are eligible. There is one rate for those aged 18–22 and another for those aged 22 and over.

Thus even quite young and inexperienced stable staff who do not necessarily fall into the category of apprentice or those undergoing training may have to be paid the minimum wage. There is very little guidance on this as yet as there have been few cases.

As an employer you must keep sufficient records to show that workers are being paid the minimum wage. These must be in a single document and must be kept for three years. The consequence for failing to keep records or pay the national minimum wage is that the employee can bring a claim to an employment tribunal for unlawful deduction of wages and recover what they should have been paid, even after they leave the job. If the worker is dismissed because of something to do with the minimum wage regulations, there may well be an unfair dismissal claim. An employer failing to keep or produce records can have a financial order made against them by an employment tribunal or the Inland Revenue, with a maximum punishment on conviction of a fine of £5000.

Working time regulations

One of the other major changes is the Working Time Regulations 1998 which came into force on 1 October 1998. Like the National Minimum Wage Regulations, these apply not just to employees but also to 'workers'. Under these regulations, working time should not exceed 48 hours over a seven day period. To calculate whether a worker is working more than this you calculate the average hours worked over a seven day period based on a 17 week period which is known as the 'reference period'. Again employers have to keep records for two years to prove that they are not exceeding the limits. It is possible for workers to agree to exclude the maximum working time regulations, but they cannot be forced to do so. Employers should not try to use any degree of force to get workers to agree, as this will both be a criminal offence and give the worker the right to claim unfair dismissal. However, even if a worker has agreed that the working time regulations shall not apply to them, they can give notice to their employer at a later date that the regulations should apply to them.

Workers are entitled to rest periods under these regulations. At the time of writing adult workers, (18 years old or more) are entitled to at least 11 consecutive hours in each 24 hour period whereas a young worker, (15 to 18 years old) is entitled to 12 hours. Adult workers are entitled to 'uninterrupted rest' of at least 24 hours in each seven day period and young workers are entitled to rest periods of at least 48 hours in each seven day period. Adult workers can be given two uninterrupted rest periods of 24 hours in each 14 day period or one uninterrupted rest period of 48 hours in each 14 day period, but this can be reduced to 36 consecutive hours where 'justified by technical or organisational reason'. Again, this might apply to say a stud where it is necessary to be on hand over the intense foaling period.

Adult workers who work more than six hours are entitled to a rest break of not less than 20 minutes, and a young worker who works more than $4\frac{1}{2}$ hours is entitled to 30 minutes. Workers employed for 13 weeks or more are entitled to four weeks paid leave which cannot be replaced by a payment in lieu except where all leave hasn't been taken and a worker leaves.

The working time regulations would not apply where the employment was such that the duration of working time was not measured or pre-determined or where the worker could determine his or her own working times. Therefore, the regulations may not apply to anyone who is in a position to organise their own working day at their own discretion.

Is this going to lead to more people being taken on on a 'self-employed' basis? Remember that just because someone is said to be self-employed, this is not conclusive proof that they are. The essence of self-employment is the element of real control by the individual over their working day. If this is absent, they may well be held to be employed.

It is also unclear just how all these detailed rules and regulations are going to be enforced. Have the Inland Revenue the time or the inclination to constantly tour the land seeking employers who have failed to keep adequate records?

Seek advice

Employment law is very complicated and although the regulations normally apply only to larger businesses and organisations, you should always take proper advice from a specialist employment lawyer if you are considering taking on staff to ensure that you are not breaching any laws or regulations. The consequences of failing to comply can include criminal prosecutions, even if you have not meant to breach any regulations, and the maximum unfair dismissal award (as at October 2001) can now be £51,700, which is a significant amount of money. You also have to take into account regulations relating to offering pensions (in particular the new 'stakeholder' pensions requirements), maternity leave and parental leave.

It is only right that workers should not be forced to work very long hours for very little pay, nor should they be under constant threat of dismissal at the employer's whim, but on the other hand horses are living animals and do require 24 hour care and supervision and so changes such as the working time regulations might affect the horse world more than some other industries.

VAT

A small but interesting point that riding school proprietors might like to consider is this. If you are both a proprietor of a school and you give lessons, the lessons you give may be VAT exempt. If you have been charging VAT you may be entitled to a rebate. VAT consultants in Prince-Martin (01673 860282) can advise further.

Chapter 2
Choosing a Riding School – and Pupils

Every riding school should be licensed, which indicates that certain standards have been met. Assuming that a school is correctly licensed, there are other factors that a potential client may want to look for in choosing a school, or additional levels of quality markers that a riding school may want to achieve.

The British Horse Society (BHS) and the Association of British Riding Schools endorsements give a level of reassurance to potential clients. A riding school will need to contact these organisations for further details of what is involved. The levels of approval for the British Horse Society are:

- A1 – Basic instruction in riding and jumping
- A2 – Instruction in riding and jumping
- A3 – Instruction up to and including BHSAI (Assistant Instructor)
- A4 – Instruction up to and including BHSII (Intermediate Instructor)
- A5 – Instruction up to and including BHSI (Instructor)
- A6 – Instruction up to and including FBHS (Fellow)

Other services offered are classified as follows:

- B – Trekking
- C – Hacking
- D – Livery
- E – Stud
- J – Riding holidays
- F – Facility centre

Choosing an instructor

One thing to watch out for when you are going to a riding school is whether your instructor is employed by the riding school or is acting as a self-employed instructor using the facilities of the riding school. If they are employed by the riding school then the riding school itself will be liable for them if they are negligent and an accident or injury occurs. If they are self-employed and just using the facilities of the riding school, then they are unlikely to be the responsibility of the riding school. You should check that they are properly qualified and have insurance before teaching you. This applies whether they are teaching you on your own horse or on a riding school horse.

The riding school will remain responsible for the safety of the premises even when the riding instructor is self-employed. This also applies to liveries. The riding school should ensure that there is a safe environment for liveries to ride in, but what they do on their own horse within that safe environment is their own affair. If, however, they are doing something clearly dangerous, they should possibly be stopped, particularly if they are presenting a danger to others.

For example, say you had an accident because although the horse you were riding was completely safe and suitable for your needs, the arena you were riding in was badly maintained causing the horse to trip and fall resulting in you sustaining an injury. The riding school would then be at fault as it would be their premises which caused the injury. If you are using a riding school horse for your lesson, even where the instructor is self-employed, it would be wise of the instructor to check that you have been provided with a suitable animal, otherwise they may be at fault for allowing you to ride an unsuitable horse. If they are giving you a lesson on your own horse, then it is unlikely that they would be at fault if an injury was caused through the behaviour of your own horse, but again it might be possible to argue that an instructor should say if they feel your own horse is unsuitable for you and too much for you to handle.

An instructor should not ask you to do something beyond your capability or what you feel confident doing, even on your own horse, but having said that, sometimes you will have to be brave in order to progress. Obviously if the instructor provides horses, then they should be safe and suitable to give the standard of lesson you require and are capable of.

It may not always be obvious whether an instructor is employed or self-employed. Sometimes, and this happens in many industries, not just riding schools or trekking centres, for legal or financial reasons staff can be expressed as being self-employed. Thus, if something did happen to you, the riding school would try to escape liability by claiming that the instructor was not employed by them. As a rough rule of thumb, the test of whether or not an instructor is self-employed is to check the level of control they have over their working environment. The greater the level of self-control, the more likely it is that they are self-employed. Can they come and go as they please, teach who they like and decline to teach others? Do they pay for the hire of the school or arena? Do they provide their own horses or are they obliged to use school horses? If the instructor has to start work at 8AM, work till 6PM and give eight lessons a day on the school horses six days a week, has a set wage and maximum holiday periods, then it may be that they are employed by the school no matter what their contract says. If a claim is made, your solicitor should check this point to make sure your claim is made against the correct person.

It can be difficult to choose a good riding school as they vary so much. It is important to stress that riding is meant to be fun and a pleasure and if you approach it with the idea that it is always going to be a disaster and result in injury, then this is the wrong attitude. Although real safety should be an important factor for you, particularly as a beginner, it is also very important to learn to ride in an atmosphere in which you feel comfortable and with an instructor who suits you. Some people do need pushing more than others, but if the instructor pushes you beyond your capability and an accident occurs, then they may be liable in negligence. On the other hand, if the instructor does not push you sufficiently, you will never progress in your riding skills. Do remember that you can always say no if you feel that the instructor is asking you do something which you do not feel safe or capable of doing.

When choosing a riding school be sure to have a look at several in the area before deciding. You will get an idea of the atmosphere of the yard just by visiting. Do the horses and stables look well cared for even if they are not all warmbloods in purpose-built stables? Does everything look neat and tidy with fencing in good condition and equipment safely put away? Is the riding school and the instructor taking an interest in you as an individual and listening to what you want to achieve from your riding, or do you feel that they will just see you as another paying customer to be put on a horse and trotted around for half an hour? Just because a school has many clients that does not necessarily mean that it is good. It may be the only school for miles around or it may be remarkably (and perhaps suspiciously) cheap. Sometimes you may say you have no choice, but should we be helping to keep bad riding schools going by this attitude? It really is worth driving that extra few miles or paying a little more to feel comfortable.

The same applies to lessons at home on your own horse. Find an instructor who suits you. There is then less chance for things to go wrong as you will be able to communicate. If you can't, find someone else. The BHS has a register of instructors and a code of conduct to which those registered should adhere. The levels of qualification (all followed by the abbreviation 'Reg'd') are:

- BHS Preliminary Teachers Certificate – BHS PTC
- BHS Assistant Instructor – BHSAI

- BHS Intermediate Teaching Test – BHS Int.T.
- BHS Intermediate Stable Manager – BHS Int.S.M.
- BHS Intermediate Instructor – BHSII
- BHS Equitation Certificate – BHS Eq.Cert.
- BHS Teaching Certificate – BHS Teaching Cert.
- BHS Stable Manager – BHS S.M.
- BHS Instructor – BHSI
- Fellow of the BHS – FBHS
- Light Harness Horse Instructor – LHHI
- Vaulting Instructor – VI
- Endurance Instructor – Endurance Instructor

There are no other distinguishing levels recognised by the BHS, but individuals with equivalent foreign qualifications may also be listed in the society's register. Those registered must attend regular refresher training courses.

Clients' riding ability

Under the Riding Establishments Act, we have seen that no-one should be allowed to hire a horse unless the licence holder is satisfied that they are competent without supervision by a responsible person. The licence holder should always do their best to decide how competent a person is. It is unfortunately not an exact science. It is not safe to rely on a new client's estimate of their own ability or to go by what they say over the telephone. Many people will say 'Oh, I've done quite a bit of riding' meaning that they have been on two trekking holidays, whereas others will underplay their ability, perhaps due to modesty or nervousness. Riders often do not like admitting they are nervous or have lost confidence, even though it happens to many people and is nothing to be ashamed of.

From a rider's point of view, if you are going to a new school or starting with a new instructor, be completely honest with the owner or instructor when booking your first lesson if you decide you like the look of the school or the instructor. If you haven't ridden for ten years and you are nervous, say so. If on the other hand you competed at Badminton Horse Trials last year, then equally you should mention that.

If you are running a riding school or are an instructor, then you should offer an assessment lesson of at least half an hour to a new client. Take the person's age, height, weight and riding experience over the telephone or when you first see them and then try to match up the most reliable horse you have with that client. If you take instructions over the telephone and then see the client and the instructions do not tally, then be ready to change the horse. If the rider is good, this will become apparent and you can move on to a horse more suited to their experience within one or two lessons. If they have a somewhat exaggerated view of their own ability and you don't move them on, then they will either accept that and start to learn, or they will think you don't recognise talent when you see it and go somewhere else and become someone else's problem. If you don't have a horse suitable for a particular client, then say so. This applies not only with regard to temperament or ability, but also to physical attributes of the horse and rider. In a legal journal in early 2001 there was a query from a solicitor acting for a client who was seeking to make a personal injury claim as a result of having suffered pelvic soft tissue injuries owing to 'forced abduction' of her hips due to riding a horse that was too wide. Those of you with overweight or wide horses may like to consider whether you are doing yourself harm in this way.

There is some debate in the horse world at the time of writing as to whether there should be a certificate of level of riding ability that a rider could take from riding school to riding school if they, for instance, move house; but there may be some difficulty with this. A rider might have a certificate saying that they can walk, trot and canter, but have they managed to do this over a period of two years on a completely unreactive horse, or have they achieved it within two or three months on a well trained and reliable schoolmaster? It is always best to make your own assessment. If in doubt put a rider on a quieter horse than you think they will need.

Riding lessons

Try and have small class sizes. Riding schools are having a difficult time with the increasing cost of keeping horses and premises, and the temptation might be to have seven or eight riders or even more in a class. This is probably too many for one instructor, who will not be able to keep control of the ride if anything goes wrong. We all know how easily one horse can set off others and if the class consists of beginners and novices, chaos can easily be the result.

Before you start a class, check the horses and riders. Is the tack fitted correctly? Are there any worn straps that might break? Are there any loose shoes that might come off or cause a horse to trip? Do the horses have any health problems likely to make them a danger – for instance a girth gall which, if irritated, might cause the horse to buck or bolt off? Do you have an elderly horse that still enjoys life but perhaps trips a lot due to stiffness? He might be suitable for use in the school, but not on the roads. Do the riders have correct riding wear? Does anyone have any injury, disability or weakness which might make it unsafe for them to ride?

The same goes for hacking out. In addition to the above, you should ensure that your riders are confident to hack out and that the horses are safe. Take all the obvious precautions that you would when hacking out yourself – wear reflective clothes, ride single-file, avoid roads where possible and in an ideal world have a leader at the head of the ride and someone to follow at the rear.

Consider the term 'responsible person' under the Riding Establishments Act. Too often lessons are given by enthusiastic but inexperienced yard helpers and this seems to be especially prevalent in classes of young children. Classes for children are often seen as 'easy' and a helper will be told to just stand in the middle and let them walk around a bit and do some exercises. But if half a dozen determined ponies decide to play up, there is little anyone can do about it, let alone a five year old rider. In particular, all this might happen under the eye of parents watching their child's lesson, so at the very least you will have unimpressed clients who may leave and go elsewhere. At worst, should litigation ensue you will be faced in court with a very angry witness who is absolutely determined that it is entirely your fault that little Belinda fell off and broke her arm. Clients will almost certainly prefer to pay for safer and properly supervised tuition on well-mannered horses and ponies, and word of mouth referrals are always the best forms of publicity.

When accidents happen

If something does go wrong, then you may want to try to resolve the situation there and then. If you are looking at this from the riding school point of view, check your insurance policy to see if you are allowed to do this. Some policies insist that no 'admission of liability' is made and if it is, the policy is void. Even an apology can sometimes be seen as an admission of liability, even though it is not. Just because you say sorry to someone does not mean that you are legally liable in negligence; that still has to be proved. You should always inform your insurers of every incident – most policies require you to do this within a certain time.

Often a senior person stepping in and restoring order, making a swift but professional apology and making arrangements for little Belinda to have two or three private lessons (assuming she is not seriously injured) at no cost, to get her confidence back, can soothe the most ruffled feathers. As always though, there is a caution. Do not let clients carry on expecting free lessons or whatever for an indeterminate period while constantly threatening 'legal action' or 'taking things further'. If you believe you were not at fault, you will just have to let them take the threatened action. If you think you were at fault, then it may be better not to offer any remedy beyond an expression of regret that an accident has happened, and supply details of your insurers.

Be careful of insisting that riders get back on the horse immediately after a fall 'before they lose their confidence'. Many of us were taught like that, but it is not generally acceptable now. Get your first-aider to check the rider over even if they seem to be all right, but be ready to call for medical help if there is any suspicion of injury. Many head injuries will not be immediately apparent. Open wounds are susceptible to infection and may require immediate attention.

If the rider is an adult you know well, the fall not severe, there are no apparent injuries and the rider is more than willing to carry on, then use common sense to judge the situation. It may be in order to carry on and there is some truth in the point mentioned above about loss of confidence. If the faller is a child, be more careful. Consult with the child's parent if he or she is there and take into account the child's wishes. If the child's parent is not there, you may prefer to end the lesson and take the child home or call their parents. A useful tip is to take personal details and contact numbers for all pupils when they begin lessons with you.

If you carry on, keep the lesson simple after a fall, perhaps shortening it a little. Do not force an obviously frightened child – or adult – back into the saddle. You could perhaps suggest they go with a helper to untack the horse and put it away so they keep in contact with the horse. Make the next lessons simple confidence-building ones.

If there is any concern or any doubt at all about the wisdom of carrying on, then err on the side of caution. End the lesson and either call for professional medical assistance or insist the injured person goes to hospital immediately, taking them there yourself if necessary.

You cannot escape liability for accidents that can be proved to be your fault by putting up a notice saying that you will not be responsible for injuries or death, howsoever caused. This falls foul of the Unfair Contract Terms Act 1977. If an injury or death can be proved to be due to your negligence, then the notice will be of no effect. You will still be liable. Similarly, getting riders to sign pieces of paper to say that they are aware that riding is risky and horses unpredictable is unlikely to help you. If you have a new rider, then you can explain this to them at their first lesson, but really it is up to you to make everything as safe as you can. A very experienced rider can to a certain extent be expected to know what the risks of riding are likely to be and to make a decision for themselves whether to accept those risks, but a new or novice rider will have little idea of what horses can actually get up to. Therefore, they cannot be said to be knowingly accepting those risks.

In terms of safety around the yard, make sure that fencing is secure and that no equipment is left lying around. Ensure that stable doors are securely bolted and that any horses that bite have a grille up. It is not sufficient to put up a notice saying 'This horse bites' as small children and animals cannot read. You are also admitting that you know that a horse has this particular problem. In an old case, *Judge* v. *Cox* (1816) (1 Stark 285) it was held that a warning not to go near a dog was indeed evidence that there was knowledge of a problem.

You may find yourself liable under the general law of negligence if one of your horses causes injury. You must take reasonable care that they don't; for instance, don't tie them up too close so that people have to squeeze behind hind legs to get through, ensure that everyone adheres to safe handling techniques, use proper leadropes in good condition and only lead one horse at a time, do not allow horses to stand unattended in the yard whilst tack is put away and ensure doors and gates have proper fastenings that open and close easily.

Instructors and staff may need to attend a Child Protection course for guidance on safe and appropriate methods for using physical contact in the course of teaching. The British Horse Society or the Association of British Riding Schools will have further information about this.

Injury caused by animals

You could also find yourself liable as the owner or keeper of a horse under the Animals Act 1971 if the horse causes an injury that falls within the circumstances and criteria set out in the Act.

A horse is classed an animal of a 'non-dangerous' species for the purpose of the Act, but the Act says at section 2(2):

'Where damage is caused by an animal which does not belong to a dangerous species, a keeper of the animal is liable for the damage, except as otherwise provided by this Act, if:

(a) the damage is of a kind which the animal, unless restrained, was likely to cause or which, if caused by the animal was likely to be severe; and

(b) the likelihood of the damage or of its being severe was due to characteristics of the animal which are not normally found in animals of the same species or are not normally so found except at particular times or in particular circumstances; and

(c) those characteristics were known to that keeper or were at any time known to a person who at the time had charge of the animal as that keeper's servant, or where that keeper is the head of a household, were known to another keeper of the animal who is a member of that household and under the age of sixteen.'

'Damage' is defined in section 11 of the Act as: 'the death of, or injury to, any person (including any disease and any impairment of physical or mental condition).

The Animals Act is not easy to interpret, but if you know that one (or more) of your horses has a peculiar habit or characteristic which could result in it causing serious injury unless prevented from doing so, then you could be liable under the Act. For instance, all horses could be said to have a tendency to kick. Most won't, but it is a 'normal' characteristic of a horse. If, however, you know that a particular horse always kicks people wearing hats, then this might be classed as a 'characteristic not normally found in animals of the same species.' In trying to decide what is a 'normal' characteristic for a 'species' you would need to compare like with like – not just whether it was normal for horses, but for that type of horse. Therefore you would need to compare Arab with Arab, Shire with Shire, etc. If a claim does arise, then usually the allegations are both under the general law of negligence and the Animals Act.

Liability is 'strict' for offences under the Act. This means in law that the fact that the incident has happened is enough for liability to arise. You do not have to have the intent that damage should be caused, nor be proved to be negligent. In the case of *Mirvahedy* v. *Henley* (*The Times Law Reports*, 11 December 2001), three horses broke out of a field and ran onto a dual carriageway, causing an accident. The field fencing was adequate and the horses owners (the defendants) were not negligent in allowing the horses to escape. It was found they had been panicked by some unknown event and escaped. The judge ruled in favour of the defendants, but the claimant successfully appealed. It was held that the accident was caused due to the normal characteristic of horses to panic in certain circumstances even if temporary. The owner only had to know the horses would behave in that way if panicked to be liable. The exceptions to this are if the damage was wholly the fault of the person suffering it or where a person voluntarily accepts the risk of the damage. However, do note that staff are not necessarily to be taken as voluntarily accepting the risk of damage just because they work with and look after the horse.

You will be a 'keeper' if you own the horse, have it 'in your possession' – generally speaking, are in charge or have control of it – or you are the head of a household where a member of that household aged under sixteen either owns the horse or has it 'in their possession'. An interesting question in this time of equality is who is going to be the 'head of the household'. The case of *Flack* v. *Hudson* (1999) (*Horse Law*, (1999) Vol. 4, Iss.4 and 6, (2001) Vol. 6, Iss. 1) makes it clear that there can be more than one keeper and that one keeper can sue another.

It is worth mentioning dogs at this point, because very often dogs and horses go together and many dogs are seen running loose around a stable yard. They may be pets, guard dogs or a combination of both.

Under the general law of negligence, the owner of an animal would be liable for reasonably foreseeable injury where they have failed to take reasonable care over the animal and that animal causes an injury. The dog or dogs concerned need not necessarily have a history of attacking people and the injury need not necessarily be caused by an attack or bite. In the case of *Draper* v. *Hodder* (1972) (2 QB 556) a child was attacked by a pack of terriers running loose. They had not been known to show any vicious tendencies previously, but the owner was still liable. In the case of *Jones* v. *Owen* (1871) (24 LT 587) two large dogs coupled together by a lead knocked into a passer-by, who fell and broke his leg, and the owner was found at fault for failing to have the dogs under proper control. There seemed no element of deliberate attack. The Animals Act 1971 applies to dogs with strange or abnormal characteristics in the same way as it does to horses.

So you need to be careful about loose dogs in a stable yard, particularly where there are children or other horses around. You should not have loose guard dogs running around for the primary purpose of protection of the premises, but it might be reasonable, for instance, to house your dog at night in the tack room as this would also have the supplementary purpose of protecting the tack. Putting up notices such as 'Our dogs bite' will not protect you and may in fact be taken as an admission that you know your dogs are dangerous.

Hazards and safety

Do not let children play on muck heaps, hay stacks or straw bales and do not stack these up too high; they can fall or topple on those trying to reach them. Muck heaps can also carry communicable diseases. Do not let young, untrained or inexperienced people use machinery, and make sure that all machinery is safe. Keep hazardous substances and medicines firmly out of the way and locked up, and securely fence off any hazards such as ponds or wells. Your riding school will be subject to health and safety legislation.

You may also be liable under the Occupiers' Liability Acts 1957 and 1984 for any injuries caused by hazards on your property. The 1957 Act applies to injuries caused to anyone who is a 'visitor' to your premises, or there lawfully. This can be someone you have actually invited there, or someone who is entitled to be on the premises. This could include your pupils if you are a riding school, the horse owners if you are a livery yard, independent instructors or trades people such as farriers attending at the premises for a purpose. It does not apply to these using the premises as a right of way.

The 1984 Act is notorious because even trespassers and burglars, who have no legal right to be there, can make a claim under it if they are injured while on your premises. This Act applies if the 'occupier' – the person having control over the premises – knows of a danger on the premises, or has reasonable cause to think that a person is or could be near the danger and should really have taken steps to prevent anyone, lawful visitor or not, being injured by that danger. A common example would be an unfenced slurry pit into which someone could fall. The occupier might escape liability, at least in part if not totally, under the Occupiers' Liability Act 1984 if a notice of a hazard or danger is very clearly worded and prominently displayed at or near the hazard such that someone reading it would know they should not go near whatever the notice warns against and that if they do so, they risk injury or death. In the case of *Staples* v. *West Dorset District Council* (1995) (PIQR 439), the defendant council escaped liability for a hazard even where there was no notice of it. The claimant slipped and fell on a wet and slippery surface and was injured. It was claimed there should have been a notice warning of this. However, the court felt that the danger was obvious to anyone anyway and therefore a notice was not necessary to warn of it.

A notice alone will not protect the occupier completely, so at the same time, practical steps such as fencing off the hazard should be put in place to actively prevent people getting anywhere near it. Fencing etc. must then be regularly checked, repaired and maintained. It is almost worse to recognise something as a hazard, fence it off and then forget about it.

The courts are not always entirely sympathetic to those injured by reason of going somewhere they shouldn't and in many cases consider that they are largely the authors of their own misfortune. But not always.

The duty under the 1957 Act in general terms is:

'to take such care as in all the circumstances of the case is reasonable to see that the visitor will be reasonably safe in using the premises for those purposes for which he is invited or permitted to be there.'

So you only have to take 'reasonable' care, you do not have to ensure that every conceivable potential hazard or danger is completely eradicated. However, the duty is likely to be higher towards children, who cannot be expected to watch out for their own safety to the same extent as adults. You should also guard against things that might be 'traps' or enticements for children. The case of *Jolley* v. *Sutton Borough Council* (2000) (*The Times*, 24 May) illustrates this. In this case, two boys were attracted to an old boat which had been abandoned and should have been cleared away by the council. While they were playing on it, the boat fell on one of them, causing serious injury. The council were held liable. Which child can resist climbing on an old tractor or up a stack of hay bales?

The duty only exists to the extent that the visitor is doing something they are permitted to do. So say, for instance, a visitor is allowed on your premises to watch a riding lesson, but they wander off away from the school and into the stabling area where they are not supposed to be and they suffer an injury there, you may escape liability if you had no reason to know they would be there.

The duty arises where:

- You are aware of a danger, or have reasonable grounds to believe it exists.
- You know or have reasonable grounds to believe that the other (i.e. your visitor) is in the vicinity of the danger, whether or not they have lawful authority to be there *and*
- The risk is one, taking into account all the circumstances of the case, for which you might reasonably be expected to offer the other some protection.

The risk can include exposure to a dangerous animal.

There have been hundreds of cases under the Occupiers' Liability Acts and while they are very interesting, each case turns on its own facts and circumstances. What may be 'reasonable' in one set of circumstances may not be in another, so the cases are illustrative but may not be wholly conclusive in any particular situation. Therefore, do not put off fencing in that rather interesting pond – do it now!

In terms of riding, ensure that all your riders are wearing properly fitted up-to-date riding hats of the appropriate safety and protection standards in force at the time. These can be checked by contacting the British Horse Society. Check that hats have not been dropped, as this could affect their strength and the protection they offer. Some riding schools provide riding hats for their customers but this is not entirely satisfactory as they may not fit correctly. It is better if the rider has their own.

Body protectors are not mandatory, but you should at least give consideration as to whether they should be used – a beginners' cross country lesson, for instance. If they are used, again they should comply with the recommended standards of protection in force at the time, which can be checked with the British Horse Society.

Riders should also have properly fitting appropriate footwear from the start – jodphur boots or long boots. Wellingtons and trainers are not acceptable. While it may be acceptable for the first few lessons for other clothing, such as jeans and sweatshirts, to be 'appropriate' rather than proper riding wear, riders should definitely be encouraged to wear correct clothing as soon as possible. It might be that your riders do not want to spend a lot on expensive riding clothes and then find they don't actually like riding, but this should not be allowed to continue indefinitely.

You should have a first-aider on staff and their name should be clearly displayed. There must be an accident book for reporting accidents and the appropriate accidents must be reported under the Reporting of Injuries, Diseases and Dangerous Occurrences Regulations 1995 (RIDDOR). The type of accidents that must be reported under these regulations are the more serious accidents, such as broken bones or death. See RIDDOR's website for the procedure for reporting accidents.

When completing the accident book it is not enough to just write 'Camilla fell off Dusty'. You should write as much detail of the incident as possible, including persons involved, description of the horse involved, time and date of the accident, the weather conditions, surface conditions, etc. Names and addresses of all involved, including witnesses, should be clearly recorded. Where relevant take photographs of injuries and the location of the accident if possible.

If your riding school is large enough to allow events, things become more complicated and health and safety standards and requirements become much more of a consideration. You may for instance need a local authority certificate for fire safety, and you may need much more extensive first-aid and medical facilities. The British Horse Society produce a number of publications and guidance leaflets for this purpose.

It must also be remembered that there is a certain level of duty on everyone to ensure their own safety. Anyone acting in a foolish or irresponsible manner, or failing to accept or adhere to instructions, whether a client, a member of staff or a member of the public, cannot expect to be able to wholly blame somebody else if by their actions they suffer an injury. If you can show that it was entirely the person's own actions that led to the injury then you may escape liability altogether. At the very least, you may be able to show 'contributory negligence' which means that you will be able to show that the person was at least partially to blame for their own injury by their own actions. Contributory negligence can be a very small contribution, or you can have 100% contributory negligence.

If you do have a difficult client, then however much you may want the income, do consider whether in the long run the cost is worth it. Is it going to be better to bite the bullet and ask the client to go elsewhere? Consider the cost, both in monetary terms and time, of becoming caught up in litigation.

Finally, as a rider, choosing a riding school and feeling safe there is a matter to a great extent of instinct and common sense. Do remember that you don't have to stay with the same riding school if you don't like it; you can move on. However, a good riding school will want to attract and keep clients and if you run a riding school there is a lot you can do to keep and maintain a safe atmosphere without too much expense. The bottom line is that riding and lessons should be a pleasure and not a matter for constant caution and worry.

Chapter 3
Deciding to Acquire Your Own Horse

There are three basic rules to remember when buying a horse:

(1) The perfect horse is out there. Unfortunately, it is perfect for some-one else.
(2) If someone seriously sets out to deceive you they will and there is very little if anything you can do to prevent it.
(3) Be prepared to walk away.

When selling a horse, the three rules are:

(1) Your horse is perfect. Except in the eyes of the buyer – when it is also overpriced.
(2) There will be at least one potential buyer who arrives with lots of friends who know even less than the buyer does. They will not buy your horse.
(3) Be prepared to refuse to sell your horse to someone if you don't think they are the right owner. You might avoid trouble later on by doing so.

The case of *Turff* v. *Light* (1997) (*Horse Law* (1997), Vol. 2, Iss. 4) nicely illustrates the third point. Mr Turff bought a horse called Bronze Knight for his 15-year-old daughter from a well known dealer, Mr Cyril Light. The purchase price was apparently in the region of £31,500 and the horse was bought as a showjumper for the girl. Unfortunately, Miss Turff fell off the horse several times and Mr Turff decided to claim against Mr Light, saying that the horse would not jump. He had paid part of the purchase price, but refused to pay the balance. The horse was sold to Germany. Evidence given in court suggested that there was nothing wrong with the horse except that it was too strong for Miss Turff: she was 'over-horsed'. An experienced rider would have had no problems with it and video evidence was supplied to this effect. Judgment was given in Mr Light's favour, but it is worth noting that the costs of the action were in the region of £50,000.

Mr Light is a businessman. He buys, sells and produces quality horses of a high standard, and if someone wants to buy one, then he is going to sell it. That is his job and partly how he makes his living. But think of the time, effort and stress he must have experienced in this litigation. Time spent seeing solicitors, discussing the matter with experts, conferring with counsel, preparing statements etc. – all time he could have been using to buy and sell horses and make a profit.

There was also the risk of losing. Because he won his case he would get the money owed to him and also his legal costs, or at least most of them, paid by the losing side. But if he had lost, he would have lost the balance of the money owed to him by Mr Turff and he would have had to pay his own and the other side's legal costs, unless he had found a solicitor willing to take the case on a Conditional Fee Agreement basis – 'no-win, no-fee'. In that situation he would have owed his solicitor nothing, but would still have been liable for the other side's costs. In practice he would have taken out an insurance policy against having to pay the other side's costs. Having won, his solicitor would have taken part of his damages towards his legal costs, in addition to the costs paid by the other side as the losers.

Most of us will not be buying and selling at that level; indeed, if a claim was made against the majority of us, it would probably be in the Small Claims Track as a claim for a sum under £5000, and no costs are awarded in this type of claim even if you win. But, for the sake of saying 'I'm sorry, I don't think my horse will suit you', is it worth the hassle? Could your bank balance stand the expense? Can your nerves stand the risk?

Horses, however much of a character we think them to be, are in the eyes of the law 'goods and chattels' and are therefore the same as a washing machine, car, sofa bed or whatever. Washing machines do, however, come with guarantees and repair warranties for when they break down. Horses usually don't. They also have a curious ability to change character overnight on change of owner, while a washing machine usually remains a washing machine after you bring it home from the shop.

One of the first things to decide is whether you want to buy a horse or try to loan one. There are good reasons, and benefits and drawbacks, for both. Loaning a horse is discussed in Chapter 7. Here we discuss buying a horse of your own.

Working out your requirements

In buying (or indeed loaning) a horse, try to protect yourself as much as you can before the purchase (or loan). Console yourself with the fact that everyone buys the wrong horse at least once (some people never buy anything else) and there is nothing you can do that will protect you 100% and guarantee you the perfect purchase or loan horse. This book is as much about preventing legal arguments as it is about how to sort them out once they arise and if you take the points in the rest of this chapter into account (but bear in mind they are not an exhaustive list), then you may at least have a great deal of useful evidence to back up your arguments if things do go wrong, or it will not be too painful to cut and run and put it all down to experience.

Are you sure you really want to own a horse and are committed to all that goes with it? If you are, be honest with yourself and a vendor as to your needs and abilities. If you are 5 ft 1 in you may *want* a 17.2 hh horse but you don't *need* one. If you buy one and he gets strong with you, it may not be that the vendor has mis-stated his well-schooled nature; it could just be that he doesn't realise someone's on his back!

Make a list of your requirements – quiet/forward going, mare/gelding, youngster/schoolmaster, native/thoroughbred, colour, cost, etc. Horses with problems are frequently cheaper, but what constitutes a problem differs from rider to rider. There is an anecdote of a visitor to a famous showjumper's yard noticing one of the top horses weaving madly. Somewhat surprised, the visitor mentioned it to the showjumper. 'I know,' said the showjumper, 'as long as he does his job in the ring, I don't care what he does in his spare time.'

When buying a horse, bear in mind that the seller does not have to tell you everything about the horse, good or bad, without being asked, but should give honest answers to specific questions. If, however, a horse has a very obvious problem, which is immediately apparent or apparent on inspection or would be if you bothered to inspect, then the vendor need not mention this at all. If, for example, a horse only has one eye, you could not buy the horse and then expect to take it back saying that the vendor did not tell you the horse only had one eye, as this would have been apparent to you anyway – or should have been. There is a story that the reason blue eyes are known as 'wall eyes' is that people would not buy horses with a blue eye, and so the vendors of such horses would always keep that side of the horse turned away from the prospective purchaser, or turned towards the wall.

Where to buy from

Buy from a trusted known source or a reputable dealer if you can. Rights and remedies differ greatly between purchasers from commercial sources and between individuals. Buying from auctions is generally reckoned to be quite risky, but in some areas of horse buying and selling it is the norm – racehorse sales for instance, but these will be attended by experienced buyers. At most large auctions there will now be facilities for pre-sale inspection and post-sale vetting, with a time limit in which to return the horse post-sale if it proves unsuitable. You would need to study the auctioneer's terms and conditions of sale carefully and see if this is available. The auctioneer will usually be selling as an agent of the vendor and anything the auctioneer says about the horse may actually be imputed to the seller.

Catalogue descriptions at auctions are generally supplied by the vendor and can sometimes amount to warranties – a sort of guarantee. Be careful if you discuss the horse with the owner prior to it going through the auction ring. The owner might say something at odds with the catalogue description or what the auctioneer has to say and what they say may override the others.

Advertisements

Look closely at advertisements. Some advertisements can contain wondrous claims for the horse but will not necessarily form a term of the eventual contract. The horse world also has its own particular language and phrases. For instance, horsy people would have a certain understanding of the phrase 'perfect gentleman' or 'genuine schoolmaster', but it is quite difficult to describe with any precision exactly what a horse so described would be like. A schoolmaster is generally thought to be a horse with a lot of experience able to teach you more than you can teach it. Factual descriptions are much easier. If a horse is described as a 15.2 hh grey gelding, then that is what it must be. It must be 15.2 hh, grey and a gelding.

You will often see advertisements that say, for instance, '100% box, shoe, catch and clip'. Has the advertiser merely forgotten the word 'traffic', or can the horse only be ridden in indoor schools? 'Forward going' – how far forward and how fast? 'Brought on slowly for the last 2 years' – why? Has it been lame for 18 months of the last two years or is it incredibly stubborn (or dim)? An advertisement has to tread a fine line between making the horse sound attractive and stressing its good points, but not making claims that are incorrect or that the horse does not live up to. Most people will take the wording of an advertisement with a pinch of salt, but it is possible for a purchaser to argue that they were induced by the wording of an advertisement to buy the horse. This is especially so if a horse is bought unseen, although this is not recommended. Advertisers should try and avoid terms such as 'potential eventer' or 'will go far in the right hands'.

It helps when selling a horse if you have photos or videos of the horse doing what you claim it can do – but as a buyer, remember the horse may have been able to do that then and with that rider, but will not necessarily be the same with you.

It will usually be apparent from the look and wording of the advertisement if the seller is a dealer or selling in some professional capacity, but if it is not, look for a 'T' at the end of the advertisement indicating 'Trade'. Also, look for one advertisement offering a number of horses, or several advertisements all apparently offering only one horse in each, but with the same address or contact numbers. The advertisers may be dealers trying to conceal the fact. You have more rights against a commercial vendor than a private one.

Vices

You will frequently see the words 'no vices'. Vices are specific bad habits or behaviour which a horse has and which may affect its health or its suitability for some types of work. They may not necessarily make it unsound. There are two old cases which define vices and unsoundness. In *Coates* v. *Stevens* (1838) (2 Mood & R 157) unsoundness was described as:

'If at the time of sale, the horse has any disease which either actually does diminish the natural usefulness of the animal, so as to make him less capable of work of any description, or which in its ordinary progress will diminish the actual usefulness of the animal, such an animal is unsound.'

A vice is described in the case of *Scholefield* v. *Robb* (1839) (2 Mood & R 210) as 'a defect in the temper of the horse which makes it dangerous or diminishes its usefulness, or a bad habit which is injurious to its health'.

So a horse with say, navicular disease, making him suitable only for light hacking, would probably be unsound, whereas rearing would be a vice, being a 'defect in the temper... making it dangerous'. A vice can however render a horse unsound – possibly a crib biter will damage its wind. A temporary unsoundness may not mean the horse is 'unsound', but it can constitute unsoundness at the time of sale. The seller may say it is curable and may even have veterinary evidence to that effect, but who knows? You pays your money, you takes your chance.

As a seller you will have to decide, when advertising, whether to disclose that the horse has a vice or other problems, or not. There is no legal requirement for you as the seller to do so at this stage, but if you do then at least your eventual purchasers cannot say they didn't know about it.

If the vice would be obvious to anyone who views or tries the horse –

chronic weaving, a severe napping problem or a physical defect for instance, then you might as well disclose it and have done with it, reflecting the problem in the price, otherwise you will waste a lot of potential buyers' time, to say nothing of your own. Be truthful. Some buyers will not in fact mind the vice. There have been cases where vices have ceased in a different environment or under a different rider. If this happens then someone will have got a bargain, but usually the seller will have disposed of a potential problem horse.

When does a vice become a vice? Does a horse count as a rearer because it reared once, twice, several times but always in the same circumstances, e.g. when frightened by a dog? Does rearing to avoid going in the trailer count? It can be difficult to decide. If a vice manifests itself after purchase, an unscrupulous seller could easily say, 'Well he never did that with me, it must be your riding/feed/lack of exercise and he will probably settle down'. It will be very difficult for the buyer to disprove this without enquiring deeply into the horse's history and gathering evidence from people who have known the horse in the past. You may find that they are reluctant to comment or get involved. If you buy from a dealer, then even the most reputable dealers can only pass on the information they have been given about a horse or that they have noticed while the horse is in the yard. If the horse has not shown evidence of a dangerous vice to the dealer, then he or she could even get round a specifically asked question, as indeed could a private seller, by saying something like 'I've never seen it do that' or 'Not to my knowledge'.

Other defects

What about the phrase 'sold as seen'? If a defect is obviously there to be seen, then you may well be assumed to have seen it, particularly if you have been given the freedom to check over the horse as you like and/or have it vetted. If it is something not obvious, even on inspection, or something only the vendor could know and hasn't said, then the phrase may not protect the vendor. The law is unclear on this point, but it is doubtful if writing these words on a receipt will absolutely protect the vendor where there is a problem with the horse that really should have been disclosed.

As a buyer, be a little wary of evasive answers. As a seller, the rule for the buyer to bear in mind may be 'caveat emptor' or 'buyer beware', but there may be some horses which are just so dangerous that they are morally not safe to sell on unless the buyer is extremely experienced and knows exactly what they are taking on and the problems are reflected in the price. In some cases it is best to have the horse put down rather than sell it on. You may even be able to claim recompense under your insurance policy if you have to do this.

Questions to ask when buying

As a prospective buyer, make a short-list of the qualities of the horse you want. Then throw it away and make a sensible list of the qualities of the horse you *need*. Look at the advertisements to make a short-list of the horses that match the requirements from your list. Telephone the ones that seem suitable in terms of height, type, cost, etc. and ask a few more questions such as what is the horse's experience, the reason for selling, how long have they owned the horse, is it presently in regular work?

Videos

Videos of horses are becoming quite a common selling tool, but do remember that they are a video of a horse at that time in a certain environment and with a certain rider, and it may not be the same for you. They can at least, however, be evidence that the horse does have the level of capability or attributes claimed.

Viewing the horse

If the horse still seems suitable, arrange to go and see it. Take a list of questions with you, as you will always forget to ask something. Below are examples of the type of questions you might want to ask, but these are not exhaustive and you must always have in mind what is important for you:

- Is there any independent evidence of the horse's age?
- Does the horse have a height/age certificate if that is important, and can you see it? It is your job to verify information of this nature and not the vet's job at the time of vetting.
- Does the horse have papers if they are important, and can you see them?
- Is the horse fully vaccinated? This may be important if you want to compete; if vaccinations are not up-to-date, you may have to start them all over again and thus there will be a delay before you can compete. At vetting, the vet will not necessarily pick up this point.
- What has the horse been doing? If the advertisement says 'Has competed at medium level dressage', when did it last do so? Are there any photos or videos available?
- Is the horse fit and ready to go, if that is what you need?

- If the horse has had a long period off, why?
- How long have the vendors had the horse and why is it being sold? Does the reason seem plausible?
- Is the horse presently insured? Has insurance ever been refused, a claim made, or are there any exclusions?
- Is it a 'loss of use' horse? Watch out for a freeze marked 'L' on the horse to indicate an insurance write-off, although not all horses are yet so marked.

Ask specific questions. 'Does he get strong when cantering out?' Try him out on this in due course. 'Is he easy to handle in the stable?' Again, test this out. Lead him in and out of the stable, pick his feet up, brush him over lightly, tack him up, etc. 'You say he is good in traffic. Do you mean he is all right with everything or are there some things he is not too keen on, tractors for instance?' Take him onto the road, but be careful.

Check that the horse really is good to catch, box, etc. by asking to see this done if possible and doing it yourself if safe to do so. Checking whether the horse is good to clip and shoe may be a little more difficult. If they are clipped neatly it is probably a good sign, but you could ask directly whether they need any sort of restraint or sedation for clipping.

Finally, you can ask the all purpose question, 'Is there anything you should tell me or that I should know about this horse that might affect whether I buy it or not?' You may be met with an amused silence. However, as a seller, if you are totally open with a prospective buyer, there is less prospect of them being able to return the horse if they discover problems later. It is not always the sellers who are the bad guys. If you know or genuinely believe that you have sold a good horse honestly described, then if someone tries to return it for what you think is a spurious or invented reason, or they threaten to sue you, you may be inclined to let them try. If you are on sure ground, you will often hear no more about it, but if they are foolish enough to pursue it, you will likely have a good defence.

Trying out the horse

As a buyer, always give the horse as much of a test run as possible before buying. Let the seller ride the horse first, so you can get an idea of whether it looks an easy ride or whether the seller looks to be struggling or riding in an unorthodox fashion. If the horse looks to be somewhat unsafe, this may make up your mind there and then without the need for you to ride. But if you do then try the horse out and there is an accident, you may not be able to make a claim against the seller, or you may be at least partly responsible yourself. Some vendors will not have facilities for you to do as much as you would like, but do not accept excuses such as, 'The saddle has gone for flocking', 'He has just had his tea and shouldn't be ridden', or 'I daren't let you out alone and I don't have anyone to accompany you'.

You are going to be handling and riding the horse and you must be satisfied that it suits your needs, or the needs of the person you are buying it for. You are looking for a willingness on the part of the seller to give you as much opportunity as possible in the circumstances available to assess the horse for yourself. This protects the seller as well. If you have been given every opportunity to satisfy yourself that the horse is what you want, there is less chance of a comeback later. Do be prepared to say thank you but the horse is not for me, if you have any doubts. There will be other horses.

Take with you an experienced person who knows your level of riding and horse experience, unless you are experienced yourself. Your riding instructor would usually be suitable. They can also act as a reliable witness to what was said and how the horse went, in case of a dispute. An honest seller may also want an independent witness available, for the same reason.

Do not turn up with your best friend who just wants to go riding on the horse. This will not bring out the best in the seller. On the other hand a seller who may have been inclined to be less than honest might be put off selling to you if you appear to be well organised, know what you want and are prepared to try the horse out thoroughly. They would prefer to sell to someone more gullible.

Unless you are absolutely sure at the time, sleep on it before you buy. Leave a deposit if necessary to reserve the horse. You may lose the deposit, but that is better than a hasty and regrettable decision.

Vetting

In all cases it is recommended that you get the horse vetted and have a blood test taken as part of the vetting procedure. It costs more but it will deter someone from selling you a horse they have drugged or sedated, and it is extremely useful evidence afterwards if you are trying to show that you were misled. Vetting is discussed in detail in Chapter 4.

Trial periods

Some sellers, private or more usually commercial, will allow a trial period, or they will allow you to return the horse within a given time for specific reasons or even if you just change your mind. Just changing your mind or deciding you don't like the colour are not legal grounds for being able to return a horse as of right. If there is nothing wrong with the horse you may only be entitled to a refund of the purchase price if there is a genuine breach of contract or the horse is unsuitable for one of the specific reasons stated. You may only be entitled to exchange the horse for another. If you return a horse and you either ask, or the owner/dealer offers to sell it on for you rather than giving you your money back or an alternative horse, do be careful. You may become legally liable to the new purchaser if something is wrong. The right to return the horse or exchange it does not affect any normal legal rights, if for instance the horse is mis-described.

If the purported sale price of the horse you exchange for is less than the price of the one you bought, you may not be entitled to the difference if there is nothing wrong with the horse you are exchanging except that you have decided it is not for you; where the price is more, you may be expected to make up the difference.

Private sellers will be more reluctant to allow a trial period, which is understandable. Trial periods can in themselves be subject to certain conditions and during the trial period you will be required to take proper care of the horse so as to be able to return it in the same condition as it came to you. In either case, private or commercial, ensure that you have appropriate and adequate insurance for the trial period, however short.

Chapter 4
Vetting Procedures

When you have decided to buy a horse, made your short-list and chosen a horse after careful questioning and trying out, you will almost certainly want to have your horse 'vetted' before making your final decision. There is no legal requirement to have a vetting carried out before purchase, but it is recommended unless you feel you are experienced enough to take a risk in not having the horse vetted, and will be able to accept any adverse consequences with equanimity. If you do not have a vetting, you may miss out on discovering a problem or two that will either make you decide you don't want the horse, or may enable you to negotiate a lower price to take the problems into account. Not having a vetting will also reduce your access to remedies. If the horse turns out to have a problem that would have been exposed at a vetting, but you chose not to have it vetted, then you are unlikely to be able to blame the seller and return the horse.

Interestingly, in the case of *van Heyningen* v. *Hoechstra* (2001) (*Horse and Hound*, 12 July; *The Times*, 7 September) where a well known show-jumper was sued over a lame mare, the purchasers did have the horse vetted before purchase – sensible move, given that the purchase price was over £300,000. The claimant's vet apparently advised them as prospective purchasers to get confirmation that there had been no previous problems and to get a written guarantee from the seller. The purchasers alleged that they were assured by two other vets and the seller that the horse did not have previous problems and that a written guarantee 'was not appropriate'. They sued the seller despite having the horse vetted. The claimants appeared to be saying that the true condition had been covered up with drugs. The court found for the claimants and awarded them compensation and legal costs totalling almost £500,000 (reported in *The Times*, 7 September 2001). It is suggested, however, that it is not safe to rely on the courts to agree with your arguments should you become involved in litigation, and if your vet makes recommendations at vetting it would probably be advisable to follow them. If you do, you may be deterred from buying a horse with a problem, but if not and there is true deception, you will be seen to have done everything you can to help yourself.

You may be tempted to miss out the vetting owing to cost. There is no doubt that it can prove expensive, particularly if you keep thinking you have found the right horse but each time another one 'fails' the vetting. There is nothing you can do about this except make your pre-purchase homework as careful as possible to try to ensure you only have genuine probabilities vetted.

The examination

Vetting is really known as the 'pre-purchase examination' and it may be worth looking at in some detail as there are a number of misconceptions about the purpose and content of the examination. In some cases there is an idea that if the horse 'passes a vet' it can somehow be taken to be perfect in every way. The examination has a specific purpose and some things will be outside its scope, although the vet, if asked, may offer a cautious comment or two. For instance, you should not expect the examination to answer such questions as 'Will the pony be suitable for my ten year old to take to camp in six months time?' or 'Is the horse 100% safe in traffic?' or 'How much can I re-sell him for?'. The vet will answer 'I can't say'. You must satisfy yourself on those points. Also, the certificate when given will only give the opinion of the vet of that horse at the particular date and time of the examination. It will not guarantee that the horse will stay like that for the next ten years, or indeed even for the next ten minutes.

A horse does not 'pass' or 'fail' a pre-purchase examination. The vet follows a certain vetting procedure and states whether they did or did not find any 'clinically discoverable' diseases, injuries or physical abnormalities. If they did, they will record them on the certificate and state whether, on the balance of probabilities, the conditions found are likely to prejudice the use for which the horse is being purchased. A horse will not be classified as sound or unsound. A horse with no problems could be said to 'pass the vet'. Equally, one with a few problems that wouldn't affect the purpose for which you were buying the horse, could be said to have passed as well. It is when the vet thinks the discovered problems may well prejudice the horse for whatever use it is meant for, that you say it fails. Even so, you can still decide to take the risk and buy the horse, but do try and negotiate a lower price. You will have no comeback if you later try to return the horse because of one of these known risks.

If the vet makes a mistake in saying that a particular problem or attribute will not prejudice the purpose for which the horse is required, and you rely on this, then you may have a claim against the vet. You would need expert evidence to show that no reasonable vet would have, or indeed could have, come to the same conclusion. The claim in these cases will be unlikely to be against the seller.

The quality and standard of the examination may vary according to the conditions under which it is carried out. Vets will do the best they can, unless it is absolutely impossible to carry out a proper procedure when the vet should refuse or ask for an alternative venue. If part of the examination is missed out for some reason, the certificate has to say so and qualify the findings. As a purchaser, you should be very careful about agreeing to miss out parts of the examination. You may have no claim later if your horse is found to be injured or to have a defect which would have shown up if the relevant parts of the examination had been done. It is also unlikely that you could claim the vet was negligent if they had fully explained to you the problems and consequences of not doing the examination or part of it and you had agreed to that.

The vet should be wary of providing a certificate on the basis of an incomplete examination and if part of it cannot be done – say for instance, there were no facilities for galloping or the weather was making it dangerous to do so – then the vet should make the problem very clear to the purchaser and his client and should perhaps even go so far as to call off the examination until proper facilities can be provided. The reason for failing to do the part of the examination should be explained clearly to the purchaser and recorded clearly in writing in the records. There are certainly shorter examination options available, but it is recommended that the full vetting procedure is carried out even if it is a little more expensive.

You should use your own vet where possible, or one recommended to you in the area where the horse is, if it is a long way from your home. The vet's duty is to the purchaser and not the vendor. The results of the vetting will be told to you, not the vendor. There is nothing to stop you as the purchaser telling the vendor why the horse 'failed' if as a result of the vetting you decide not to buy. The vendor may be totally unaware of a problem and may be pleased to have it brought to their notice – or they may be annoyed that they have been found out. When looking at a horse with a view to purchase, it may be as well to ask whether the horse has ever failed an examination and why. The reason may not bother you. For instance, a horse with a sarcoid may fail, but you might be happy to take the horse on and might be willing to try to deal with the problem. You might be able to negotiate a reduction in price to allow for this.

Veterinary records

With regard to the horse's previous health history, veterinary records are of great value and a vendor who has nothing to hide should have no problem in producing them for the vet if asked. If the vendor refuses, or does not wish to answer questions about the horse's previous history, then you or the vet should perhaps question why. Veterinary records are confidential to the owner and neither you nor the vet at this stage can insist on them being available, although they might become what are called 'disclosable documents' during the course of any litigation.

A disclosable document is one which is relevant to the issues in a case and which both sides and the court should see and indeed have a right to see, as the document will or is likely to have useful information relevant to a case, whether it be to the good or detriment of either party. There is another type of document used in court cases, called 'privileged' documents. An example of a privileged document would be an expert's report prepared at your request. The other side has no automatic right to see privileged documents, although sometimes a court can order that they should be produced. Therefore, if you were for instance, making a claim against a vet and you had a report which said that the vet was not negligent, you need not use that report by showing it to the other side. You might want to obtain another report which supported your claim. You could use that one by showing it to the other side as it supported your case.

There can sometimes be arguments over what is and what is not a disclosable or a privileged document. This can only be resolved by applying to court to get the court to make a ruling as to whether the document, or indeed other forms of evidence, do have to be shown to the other side – disclosable – or whether they can remain confidential to you – privileged.

With regard to vet's records, if someone is alleging, for instance, that you have sold them a horse with a long-standing problem such as laminitis, you may willingly want to show them your horse's vet's records so they can see there is no record of the horse having laminitis while it was with you. Strictly speaking, such a record would only show that the horse was not *treated* for laminitis while it was with you, but no responsible horse owner would allow a serious condition to go untreated and so it would be likely to show up in a record if it had occurred. You could argue therefore that you did not sell a horse with a laminitis problem because you didn't know it had one, or that the laminitis has arisen since the sale.

The records are unlikely to show the horse's history prior to the last owner. A horse may therefore have had laminitis with a previous owner, and the immediate past owner has just been lucky. You do not know whether the immediate past owner was told of the laminitis problem and if they maintain they were not, then you may be in difficulty in making a claim. You would really need the horse's entire veterinary history and this could be both time-consuming and expensive. Some past owners may not give their consent to the records being made available. Again, to a large extent it will depend on the economics of a claim. As a general rule, the bigger the potential claim and the more important it is, the more expense can be justified.

Choice of vet

The vet could be confronted with an ethical problem if you buy a horse locally and it turns out that you and the vendor have the same vet. If the vet knows that the horse you are trying to buy does have particular problems, or a particularly difficult history, he or she will usually try to obtain the consent of the seller to reveal the past history and should not examine the horse if the consent is not forthcoming. The vet would have a dilemma. If he or she examines the horse knowing that it has had a latent defect, i.e. one that would not be immediately apparent on inspection, for the vet not to mention this would be professionally unethical even though there may be no obligation on the seller to bring it to your attention. But the vet would not have the consent of the owner to mention it, so may not be able to do so.

On the other hand, do not assume just because the vet says he or she would prefer not to examine the horse, that there is something wrong with it. The vet may just be being prudent in avoiding an obvious conflict of interest from the start. Don't have a horse vetted by the seller's own vet; it can cause all sorts of professional and ethical difficulties.

Before the examination

Before the examination, the vet should ask you as the purchaser what you want the horse for and why you have chosen this particular horse. He may confirm with you that you have satisfied yourself that it is suitable and that your purchase now largely depends on a favourable vetting and a final decision.

Tell the vet if you are a complete novice and inexperienced. The vet should ask you whether you are aware of the limitations of the examination and that the examination will not necessarily be suitable for insurance proposal purposes. An insurance company may require an additional examination before or after purchase depending on when your insurance is to run from.

Before a pre-purchase examination the horse to be examined must:

- Have its identification documents available. Freeze mark and brand documents are also useful.

- Be capable of being 'handled', i.e. allow its feet to be picked up, its teeth to be looked at, or whatever.
- Be able to be lunged on both reins.
- Be properly shod or have its feet trimmed so that it can move freely without the risk of injury.
- Be brought in and stabled for at least two hours prior to examination and not have been exercised on that day.

The vendor's consent must be obtained if a blood test is requested and the most appropriate time to do this is when the appointment time for the examination is being made. If the vendor refuses, the vet should really consider why.

The examination procedures

The pre-purchase examination is in five stages. The vet will work through the procedure either writing down his findings or using a worksheet. It is recommended that you attend the vetting examination. The five stages are: preliminary examination, trotting up, strenuous exercise, rest, and trotting up again and feet.

Preliminary examination

The vet is likely to have a general look over the horse and get an overview. The horse should not be tacked up at this point. The vet will be getting an overall impression of whether the horse looks generally in good condition and well kept with no obvious deformities, injuries or diseases. The vet might, for instance, note the bedding. Is the horse on shavings because of a straw allergy or because the owner prefers it? Is there evidence of any vice – for example, heavily chewed woodwork can indicate crib-biting. Is the horse standing square – weight on the hind feet can indicate laminitis.

Having gained an initial impression, the vet will then fully examine the external parts of the horse, checking its limbs, eyes and skin and listening to its heart. Its teeth should be checked. Handling the horse in this way can also given an indication of its temperament. Does it seem bothered or upset by the attention or does it seem to be enjoying the fuss? Is it possibly suspiciously quiet?

Trotting up

The horse is usually walked up and back and then trotted up and down in the same way on a loose rein. It may then be circled both ways and backed up for a few steps. Flexion tests are done. A hard flat surface is usually required for this part of the procedure as uneven or slippery surfaces can give a wrong impression.

Strenuous exercise

This can be done by riding or lungeing the horse, but a note should be made of whichever is used. The vet should watch the tack being put on in case this suggests problems. When the horse is sufficiently loosened up or warmed up it will be required to gallop. This should show up any breathing difficulties such as roaring. The vet will also check the heart rate.

Rest

The horse will be rested for about half an hour. This is the boring part during which time you might like to do a crossword or something.

Trotting up again and feet

The horse will be trotted up again as before to see if it has developed any lameness or stiffness. The vet will also test the feet for balance and symmetry and for any soreness or defects, boxy feet, uneven feet, corns, etc. The vet will undoubtedly note the shoeing and can ask any questions about slightly unusual shoes, heartbar shoes for instance.

The vet may then take a blood sample if requested and with consent. This will be stored for a time in case a dispute arises and if so, it will be tested on payment of a fee.

Other matters

If you want any 'extras' such as x-rays, endoscopic examination, preg-nancy tests, etc, then you should make this clear prior to examination so that you can obtain consent and the vet can have the necessary facilities available or arrange to have the horse in a clinic to do them. Such pro-cedures do have their limitations and the vet should explain these to you.

The vet will then probably have a chat with you generally about his or her findings and will either give you the report then or will go away to prepare it. The vet should take care to fill in the form properly and fully. In the case of *Leer* v. *Griffiths* (1996) (*Horse Law* (1997) Vol. 2, Iss. 2) it was found that a vet had filled in a vetting form in a careless manner and had probably missed a lameness by omitting to see the horse ridden or worked. Vets will usually be following the 'Twelve Principles of

Certification', which is guidance on vetting procedures set out in the veterinary professional conduct rules. If there are any doubts, the vet may advise at this stage whether further tests or examinations are necessary. All information relative to the pre-purchase examination will be kept by the vet usually for a period of about seven years before destruction.

Although it is the vet's job to conduct a pre-purchase examination with reasonable care and skill and to give you an opinion on the horse's suitability for its purpose, within the parameters of the test, ultimately it is your decision as purchaser as to whether to buy the horse or not.

Chapter 5
Buying the Horse – the Legal Part

Assuming the horse has received a favourable vetting report and you have decided to buy the horse, you will be on the verge of entering into the contract to buy it.

Contracts for sale

A contract for sale is described in section 2(1) of the Sale of Goods Act 1979 as a contract by which the seller transfers or agrees to transfer the property in goods to the buyer for a money consideration called the price. If there is no 'consideration' then there is no legal contract of sale. The horse may still change hands, but it may then be a gift. The 'consideration' need not be in money, it can be in kind, but an exchange of, say, two horses does not constitute a sale. Contracts for sale can be absolute or conditional and the sale is only complete where under the contract of sale the 'property' in the goods is actually transferred from the seller to the buyer. 'Property' is a legal concept and does not necessarily mean the actual physical property, in this case, the horse. It is more the idea of the transfer of legal ownership. Thus, the actual horse could for some reason be handed over to the buyer before all the formalities of sale were complete, but the property would not be transferred until they were complete. The horse in those circumstances might be in the buyer's possession, but would not actually be owned by the buyer until the formalities of sale were complete.

Do remember that contracts are not only made under the Sale of Goods Act. They can be made under what is called 'common law', that is, law that exists but is not necessarily written down in a statute such as the Sale of Goods Act. Private individuals can make a contract between themselves where the requirements are met for a contract to exist of offer, acceptance and consideration.

Where the transfer of the property and the goods is to take place in the future or is subject to some condition to be fulfilled later, then the contract is called an 'agreement to sell'. You want the horse, therefore you will make an offer to purchase to the seller. This may be at the asking price or less, or possibly more if there is a lot of competition. If the seller accepts your offer then there will be a legally binding contract. This will not necessarily mean that a written document called a contract is drawn up. Contracts can be, and frequently are, merely oral. What counts is that a legal relationship has been entered into. You then purchase the horse at the appropriate time in the future and/or when the required condition is fulfilled. If the condition is not fulfilled, then you may not be obliged to go through with the purchase.

As mentioned above, contracts for sale can be in writing or made orally or partly in writing and partly by word of mouth. In some cases there may be a written contract, perhaps in standard terms but this can be varied deliberately or accidentally by what is said verbally (*Couchman* v. *Hill* (1947) (1 KB 554, 1 All ER 103) Some contracts can be implied, that is, all the formalities of a contract may not be expressed to you, or not expressed very clearly, but nevertheless, by the circumstances and the actions of the parties, a contract is entered into, or is expected to be entered into. Many contract claims arise out of the confusion of one or more parties as to exactly what they are doing and one or more of the parties can often be mistaken as to what is being done. Such claims can be extremely tortuous to unravel and in many cases much will depend on just who did or said what. Do be clear about whether you want to enter into a contract or not. Do not, for instance, say something like 'Yes, I'll take him, but can I just think about it overnight? Either you've decided you want the horse, in which case you say 'Yes, I'll take him', or you want to think about it in which case you say 'Can I think about it overnight and give you a firm answer tomorrow?'. The seller does not necessarily have to give you extra time, of course, particularly when there is a lot of interest.

An often quoted example of a contract being entered into without either party stating their wishes expressly is where you go into a restaurant and order a meal. You would not have to state specifically to the restaurant that you wished to enter into a contract to purchase a meal and would the restaurant be prepared to accept your offer. Neither would you expect a waiter to appear with a written contract for you to sign before you order. It is implied by the circumstances that there is, or will be, a contract as this is what normally happens in restaurants and you have ordered a meal and the restaurant has then gone on to supply it. You could not legitimately refuse to pay for your meal by saying that you didn't realise you were entering into a contract with the restaurant, or that you didn't intend to enter into a contract. The contract is implied by all the circumstances.

You cannot make a contract with a minor child so do not under any circumstances negotiate or try to make a contract with a minor or rely on any assurances they give. It can sometimes be difficult to gauge someone's age, but if in doubt, ask to speak to their parents or 'someone in charge' and if you can't, then go no further.

At auction, the contract is made at the fall of the hammer after the final bid is accepted and there is usually no way out unless the auctioneer's terms of business allow for the remedying of mistakes or the return of the horse within a specified time for specified reasons. Read the terms and conditions of each individual auctioneer carefully before the sale as there may be differences between auctioneers or even different types of sale.

Once your contract is made you must go through with it unless something intervenes to render the contract unenforceable or not capable of being completed. For instance, you might enter into a contract to buy a certain horse, but not necessarily go to see it. It might be a horse you know well and have been trying to buy for a while. Unbeknown to both the buyer and the seller, the horse has died before the contract was even made. There is no suggestion that the seller intended to mislead the buyer for these purposes. The contract is void, i.e. it doesn't exist. It is impossible to fulfil. If on the other hand the horse sadly dies ten minutes after your contract has been completed, then you as buyer may well have to bear the loss.

As a further example, if both you and the seller are genuinely mistaken as to what is being bought and sold, then you can both withdraw in certain circumstances from the contract as if it had never been made. Sometimes, after you discover the mistake you may still be happy to go through with the sale and you may or may not be entitled in some circumstances to some level of compensation or price adjustment to compensate for any loss caused by the mistake.

An example of this might be if the buyer thought he was buying a well known showjumper, but was in reality buying a horse of a similar name, but without the same level of ability. The seller thinks he is selling the horse the buyer wants. The mistake is later discovered, but by now the buyer is fond of the horse and it is beginning to come on nicely, so the buyer is prepared to keep it. There has been a genuine mistake (as opposed to a misrepresentation, where one party misleads the other so as to induce them into the contract) so technically there is no contract. The seller could take back the horse, or the buyer could keep it if agreement is reached, with a possible price adjustment. If the mistake actually makes no difference to the buyer and the seller, then the contract is likely to be held to remain in existence.

If you enter into an agreement to buy a horse 'subject to a satisfactory vetting' then your contract is not completed until the vetting has been done and the horse is pronounced suitable for you to buy. The horse still in effect belongs to the seller until this happens. If on the other hand you decide to buy the horse there and then and take it away with you, then your contract will be made immediately. As buyer or seller, check that you are still insured even when a sale is not quite completed, and as a buyer check that you are insured from the moment of purchase.

If your contract for sale is subject to a future condition which is fulfilled, then you may have to go ahead with the contract even though you have changed your mind for some other unconnected reason. If on the other hand the condition is not fulfilled, you may not have to go ahead with the contract.

Rights to sell

You cannot sell something you do not own as you cannot comply with a legal procedure called 'passing title'. If you have 'legal title' to something, this means in effect that it is yours in law – you own it. You will have heard of 'title deeds' to a house. Horses do not have title deeds, though some will have 'papers' which will be, for instance, evidence of their breeding, their age, or perhaps their height. Such 'papers' do not prove that the person selling the horse has the right to do so. The papers could be stolen, as could the horse. The papers usually just tell you something about the horse.

In order for a horse to legally become someone else's, 'title' has to pass to the new owner. If you do not have 'title ' in the first place, you cannot pass it on and the new owner may not in fact own the horse. The rightful owner, the one with the ability to pass title, could come forward and either ask for the horse back or get a court order ordering the return of the horse to them on the grounds that title has not passed. There can be situations where the buyer would be entitled to argue that they quite reasonably thought that the person selling the horse had every right to do so and was in fact capable of 'passing title', and therefore they should be entitled to keep the horse. It is similar to situations where contracts can be implied by the circumstances and the actions of the parties.

This area of law is extremely complex and whole books have been written on the law of 'agency' as it is known. It would be impossible here to explain the law in any detail, but a relatively simple example, in terms of circumstances if not in law, can be given. Stephanie owns a horse, Jack. Jack is kept at livery with Emma. Stephanie works long hours and cannot get to see Jack very often. Without Stephanie's knowledge, consent or approval, Emma decides to sell Jack. She does not own him, so can't pass the title. Also, of course, she has no right or authority to sell him.

Catherine sees Jack advertised and makes an appointment to go and see him. She has to travel a fair way and knows nothing about the yard where he is kept, nor does she know Stephanie or Emma. Emma seems very pleased to show Jack off to her and knows a lot about him and his history (he has been in her yard for five years but of course Emma does not tell Catherine that he is a livery). While Emma doesn't actually say that she owns him, Catherine has no reason to doubt that she does. In fact, the thought that Emma may not own him doesn't even cross her mind. There seems nothing unusual or suspicious about the sale. Catherine likes Jack very much and agrees to buy him there and then. She picks him up the next day, pays the asking price and returns home delighted with her new horse.

Stephanie comes into the yard a week later, having been on a business trip abroad, and finds that Jack is not there. Emma explains that she has sold him as she thought Stephanie had lost interest, but he has gone to a very good home. Stephanie is quite rightly furious and wants Jack back. She tells Emma that she had no right to sell him and therefore the new 'owner' does not in fact own him. She wants him back and tells Emma that she will have to give Catherine the purchase price back. Emma offers her the purchase price instead of Jack, but Stephanie does not want this. She wants her horse back. The question is whether she is going to be able to achieve that.

Regrettably, the answer is not going to be clear. Emma certainly had no right to sell Jack and cannot 'pass title'. So Catherine may not be the rightful owner; Stephanie may still be. Catherine may be entitled to argue that due to the circumstances in which she bought Jack, it would not have been reasonable for her to ask specifically whether Emma actually owned Jack, as everything pointed to the fact that she did and that she had the right to sell him. Emma did not tell her that there was a third party involved and she thought she was dealing with Emma. Therefore, to her mind, she has a contract with Emma, title has passed and she should be allowed to keep the horse. Even if Stephanie goes so far as to apply to court to obtain an order forcing Catherine to give Jack back to her, Catherine could then argue that the court should really order that she can keep Jack, and Stephanie should just be entitled to financial compensation for her loss, i.e. the purchase price should be hers, not Emma's. If the court ordered that Catherine could keep Jack but would have to pay compensation to Stephanie instead, then in turn she would want to claim against Emma for the return of the purchase price – the amount she has had to give to Stephanie.

A court may order that she should give the horse back, title not having passed. Stephanie may not necessarily be responsible for paying Catherine her purchase price back and in that case Catherine would have to look to Emma for that.

Emma might want to argue that she thought she had permission to sell the horse. In the circumstances set out above, that would be unlikely, but sometimes people can make mistakes and honestly believe that they have authority to do something. This would not make any difference in law. If a person professes to contract as an agent for another person, then they are saying to the person relying on that authority, i.e. the purchaser, that they do have the authority they profess to have, even if they don't say so expressly (*Collen* v. *Wright* (1857) (All ER 8 E&B 647).

If Emma had genuinely been acting as Stephanie's agent and Stephanie had wanted to sell Jack, then Emma would have had authority to sell Jack, but the contract would have been between Stephanie and Catherine. If Catherine wanted to return Jack, or if there was some breach of contract, she would have to negotiate with Stephanie, not with Emma, although all her negotiations had been with Emma. Catherine would not have a contract with Emma.

In some cases, a relatively new law, the Contracts (Rights of Third Parties) Act 1999, gives third parties rights to enforce terms of contracts where they would not have had that right before. Usually, only the parties to the actual contract can, for instance, enforce or vary a term of a contract. This Act extends some rights to others, even where they are not actually parties to the original contract. This is quite a specialised area of law and beyond the scope of this book to explain in detail. You will need to take specialist legal advice if you think this situation might apply to you.

Because the law in this area is complicated, you really would need to take proper legal advice on the exact circumstances of your particular situation. The example above only serves as an illustration of possibilities. Basically, if the horse is not yours don't sell it or even try to.

As an owner you can give someone authority to sell your horse on your behalf, but if you do so the person selling should obtain your clear instructions in writing, including any special instructions such as minimum selling price, and should stick to them absolutely. Leave a contact number or address for last minute negotiations and both parties should make a note of any altered instructions and the date and the time they were given. Making notes of things as they happen is generally a good idea in any circumstances.

There is a safeguard for people buying as a consumer, that is as a non-business or private buyer, from a business, i.e a dealer. Under section 12(1) of the Sale of Goods Act 1979 there is an implied term on the part of the seller 'that in the case of a sale he has a right to sell the goods, and in the case of an agreement to sell he will have such a right when the property is to pass'. This is so unless the contract of sale falls within section 3 of the Act, which says that where it appears from the contract or can be inferred from the circumstances that the seller only intends to pass whatever title they or a third person do have, then the implied term is invalid and there is no implication under section 12(1).

Usually handing over the purchase price will be enough to seal the agreement. Some people think that it is lucky to return a small part of the purchase price to the buyer or hand over a piece of silver money to the seller on taking over the horse. It might work!

Sale of Goods Act

Horses are goods and as such are subject to the Sale of Goods Act 1979, as amended by the Sale and Supply of Goods Act 1994. The important point about this is that the Act *only* applies where one person sells in the course of business while the other person is a consumer, i.e. a non-commercial or private buyer. When you are looking through advertisements for your horse, dealers and commercial enterprises should be obvious from the text, or there should be a 'T' for trade at the end of the advertisement where otherwise it looks like a private sale.

You do not have to have a big sign over your door saying 'dealer' to be one. The court can decide that you are a dealer if there is a history, sometimes even a very short one, of a 'course of dealing' with horses and ponies by buying and selling them with some element of repetition or regularity, usually making a profit. Every dealer has to sell a first horse. There are others who genuinely have large families which rapidly grow out of ponies and have to change them often. They would not necessarily be held to be dealers. There is no hard and fast rule as to what constitutes a commercial trader. Even if you ask an outright question such as 'Are you a dealer/expert selling commercially?' you may get the answer 'Oh no, I am just selling this one for a friend who has left to live in Australia' or whatever.

The Act does apply to someone selling as an agent for someone else, but not when the person they are selling for is not a business and you as the buyer either know that, or the agent has taken reasonable steps to bring it to your notice before the contract. Thus, if the dealer is selling a horse that they themselves have bought and own, the Act will apply because the dealer is in effect selling their own horse. If the dealer is selling the horse on behalf of a private owner and this is made clear to you, then the Act probably will not apply.

The general rule is that the contract of an agent is the contract of the principal, but this is not always the case. An agent is basically someone with authority to act on behalf of someone else in making a contract and binding them to that contract. It is a very complicated area of law and you can find that some sales go through several tiers of agent and possibly have more than one owner involved. Sometimes the agents are just go-betweens and can neither enforce the contract they have made, nor be liable for anything that goes wrong; in other cases there can be liability on the part of an agent, particularly when they are acting outside the authority given to them by the ultimate owner or principal, or where they do not reveal the fact that they are acting on behalf of someone else and it is not obvious from the circumstances of the sale. It all depends on the exact circumstances of each transaction. You would need to take more detailed legal advice if you became caught up in a dispute involving various agents and principals.

The Sale of Goods Act, and Trade Descriptions Act 1968, not only apply to horses being sold in the course of business but also to equipment sold in the course of business, i.e. tack, rugs, etc. The Sale of Goods Act has a useful section for buying by sample. This might apply when you are buying hay or straw, where you are unable to check every bale but the seller shows you a sample. There is an implied term under the Act that the 'bulk of the goods ordered will correspond to a sample in quality and that they will not have any default making them unsatisfactory which would not be apparent on reasonable examination of the sample'.

The Sale of Goods Act is generally thought to give rise to a lot of grey areas and there may be no straight or definitive answer to the question of whether you can or can't return a horse or equipment and get your money back. If you think that you have a genuine complaint, and the seller is not prepared to exchange the horse or give you your money back, then your only option may be formal litigation, often in the Small Claims Track if your claim is worth £5,000 or less, or in the County or High Court if more. The exception to the £5,000 limit in the Small Claims Track is if your claim is for or includes a claim for a personal injury and the injury is 'worth' £1,000 or more. Then your claim can be heard in the County or High Courts.

Litigation concerning horses can, however, often involve very large sums of money, particularly for specialist horses such as showjumpers or dressage horses. In the case of *van Heyningen* v. *Hoechstra* mentioned in Chapter 4, a well known showjumper was sued for over £60,000 over a mare that had originally had a sale price of £350,000. It was alleged that the mare went lame owing to a pre-existing problem, which was denied by the seller. It was somewhat surprising that even with a history of lameness, the mare still had an alleged value of £200,000, although this was disputed and required a further hearing to resolve. The claim was basically for the difference in value of the mare with and without the history, taking into account the fact that the full purchase price had never been handed over.

Implied terms

One of the important factors of the Sale of Goods Act is that it implies various terms into contracts. Implied terms are such terms as are held to be in every agreement by law, even where the agreement does not specifically say that the term is there. The alternative to an implied term is an express term – one that is expressly stated to be incorporated in and form part of the contract. Implied terms are there for protection, usually of the non-commercial buyer, and they cannot be excluded. Beyond this, the express or stated terms of a contract can be more or less as the parties agree. Once the contract is made, one party cannot change the terms 'unilaterally' – that is, without the agreement of the other party or parties.

One of the first terms implied by the Sale of Goods Act is that the seller has the right to sell the horse (or indeed any goods) and that there are no 'encumbrances' on either the horse or the goods, such as, for instance, an outstanding hire purchase agreement which hasn't been paid off. Rights to sell were discussed earlier in this chapter.

There is an implied term that the goods will correspond with their description. Let's say you choose to buy a 17.2 hh chestnut gelding over the telephone going only by his description, and the horse when delivered is in fact a 16 hh grey mare. You can send it back because it is not in accordance with its description. Telephone buying of course is not recommended.

Section 14 of the Act gives implied terms with regard to the quality of the goods, or in this case the horse and its fitness for the purpose required. This is the part of the Act that is most open to interpretation and which gives rise to most litigation. It would not be possible here to state all the possible permutations of when a horse might or might not be of 'satisfactory quality' and generally 'suitable for the purpose' for which you are buying it. It is worth, however, setting out the wording of this section of the Act:

Section 14(1)

'Except as provided by this section and Section 15 below [refers to sale by sample] and subject to any other enactment, there is no implied term about the quality or fitness for any particular purpose of goods supplied under a contract of sale.'

This means that only the items mentioned in the Act can be automatically implied. Anything else you will have to ask specifically about.

Section 14(2)

'Where the seller sells goods in the course of a business, there is an implied term that the goods supplied under the contract are of satisfactory quality.'

Section 14(2A) explains 'satisfactory quality':

'For the purposes of this Act, goods are of satisfactory quality if they meet the standard that a reasonable person would regard as satisfactory, taking account of any description of the goods, the price (if relevant) and all the other relevant circumstances.'

The test is not necessarily whether you regard the goods as satisfactory, but whether a hypothetical reasonable person would do so. Section 14(2B) says:

'For the purposes of this Act, the quality of goods includes their state and condition and the following (among others) are in appropriate cases, aspects of the quality of goods:

(a)   Fitness for all the purposes for which goods of the kind in question are commonly supplied.
(b)   Appearance and finish.
(c)   Freedom from minor defects.
(d)   Safety.
(e)   Durability.'

This particular section gives an idea of the things the law will take into account but it should not be regarded as definitive. Basically speaking, it is saying that you get what you pay for.

Section 14(2C) says:

'The term implied by subsection 2 above [implied term that the goods are of satisfactory quality] does not extend to any matter making the quality of goods unsatisfactory:

(a)   Which is specifically drawn to the buyer's attention before the contract is made.
(b)   Where the buyer examines the goods before the contract is made, which such examination ought to reveal.
(c)   In the case of a contract for sale by sample which would have been apparent on reasonable examination of the sample.'

Thus, if a seller does draw your attention to a particular defect which might otherwise render a horse or piece of equipment of unsatisfactory quality, then you cannot go back later and make a claim based on that defect. If it is drawn to your attention and you nevertheless accept the horse or equipment with it, then you will be deemed to have accepted the defect. For example, this would apply to a saddle with a mark on it, a rug with a slight tear or a horse with a vice made known to you.

Section 14(3)

'Where the seller sells goods in the course of a business and the buyer expressly or by implication makes known to the seller any particular purpose for which the goods are being bought, there is an implied term that the goods supplied under the contract are reasonably fit for that purpose, whether or not that is the purpose for which such goods are commonly supplied except where the circumstances show that the buyer does not rely or that it is unreasonable for him to rely on the skill or judgement of the seller or credit broker.'

It is under section 14(2B) that you may have a remedy if, for instance, you say to a dealer that you are buying a horse for a specific purpose, i.e. as a showjumper, a hunter or as a novice ride. The dealer or seller assures you that the horse complies with your requirements and you rely on the seller's assurance in purchasing that horse. If you do not rely on the seller's assurance but make up your own mind anyway, or it would be unreasonable for you to say that you relied on the seller's or dealer's skill, then you may not succeed in a claim under this head. It might therefore be unreasonable for a top class professional three-day event rider or show-jumper to try to escape a contract by saying that they relied on the seller's skill and judgement in saying that a horse was fit for its purpose, as given the right facilities they are perfectly capable of assessing the horse themselves and making their own decision. However, a novice rider or someone experienced in riding but with no experience or skill in choosing say, a dressage horse, might be able to rely on the fact that they made their requirements known to the seller and relied on their word.

Be careful if buying in Scotland, where the Sale of Goods Act does not apply.

Chapter 6
Misrepresentations and Warranties

Misrepresentation

If you buy privately, your rights and remedies are severely restricted as the Sale of Goods Act will not apply where both parties buy and sell as individuals. Neither will the Trade Descriptions Act, which applies to items misdescribed in the course of trade and is more suited to inanimate objects than horses. You will have to rely on proving that the seller had 'misrepresented' the horse to you and that you entered into the contract on the basis of what has now turned out to be a misrepresentation. It can be very difficult indeed to prove misrepresentation as the seller can always maintain that the change in the horse's behaviour or whatever occurred after the sale and they had no evidence or knowledge of the problem while the horse was with them.

Similarly with a disease such as navicular. The horse may go lame within a week or so of you buying it and is then discovered to have navicular disease. Your vet may maintain that there is no way that the seller could not have been aware of a problem with the horse, as the navicular must have been quite long-standing. This is something that perhaps should have been picked up in a pre-purchase examination, but may not have been without x-rays or scans and, of course, they are not part of the usual vetting procedure. There may have been no indication that an x-ray might be needed. If in this situation you could get hold of the horse's previous veterinary records and show that the vet had indeed been called out to suspected or actual navicular then you may have a claim, but the difficulty is in getting hold of the records. They are confidential to the owner.

If the seller has merely turned a blind eye to the fact that the horse may have something seriously wrong with it and has just decided to get rid of it without trying to identify the problem, then it would be much harder to make a successful claim as there would be nothing in the records even if you could get them. The seller may in fact be innocent of the fact that the horse has a long-standing problem.

There are three types of misrepresentation:

(1) *Innocent misrepresentation.* This is where there is a misrepresentation
but the seller honestly thought that what he or she was saying was
true and had no reason to think it wasn't. If as the buyer you can
prove this, then you may be able to 'rescind' the contract, i.e. over-
turn the contract as if it had never been. You give the horse back and
you get your money back. In some specific circumstances damages
may be awarded, even where the misrepresentation was innocent.
For this to happen, there would need to be some sort of 'special
relationship' between the parties giving rise to a 'duty of care', or
there may be a 'statutory right' – a right by law – to damages. You
would need to take specific advice as to whether these existed in the
circumstances of your particular purchase.

(2) *Negligent misrepresentation.* Here again there is a misrepresentation
but the seller makes it carelessly without really thinking about it, or
has no reasonable grounds for thinking that the statement is true. In
these cases you as the seller can be negligent if you make a statement
which, if you had bothered to make enquiries, you would have
found was untrue or misleading. You could also be at fault as a seller
if you make a statement about the horse while thinking 'that can't
possibly be true – oh, well, it's not for me to question it'. Negligent
misrepresentation is not entirely innocent, but at the same time there
may have been no definite intention to mislead. Where there is a
negligent misrepresentation there is often a right to both recission of
the contract and damages if appropriate.

(3) *Fraudulent misrepresentation.* This is where the seller actively seeks to
mislead by making a false statement. It can also be a criminal offence.
If you discover you are the victim of a fraud, you can withdraw from
the contract completely or you can choose to go ahead with it and
claim any damages due. You can't do both, though if the matter got
as far as court, you could ask for both in the alternative if you didn't
mind which.

You might, for instance, buy a stallion believing it to be a certain
very well-bred horse, and pay a lot of money for it. It later turns out
that you have been fraudulently sold a completely different but similar looking horse of no pedigree or value. You can choose to return
the horse and try and get your money back, or if you have become
fond of the horse, you could choose to keep him and claim damages
– possibly the difference between the price you paid and what the
horse might be worth. In addition, you might be able to claim for
future lost income that the well-bred stallion you thought you were
buying would have generated.

Be aware that if someone actively sets out to defraud you there is very little that you can do to protect yourself. They are likely to have set the fraud up very plausibly.

The representation will be false if it is false both in 'fact and substance' and the falsehood exists at the time the representation is made. The person to whom the representation is made must take some action as a result of the representation – usually this will be the decision to buy.

You could ask for some sort of assurance in writing from the seller, but there are problems with this. A genuine seller may be happy to give one, but equally may be indignant that their word is not good enough and may refuse. A dishonest seller won't give one or will only give one so vague that it can't be relied on for anything. If after all your careful investigations you are pinning your hopes of successfully buying the right horse on a sheet of paper, you may be disappointed.

Warranties

Is there anything you can rely on when buying a horse? No. The nearest you might get is a warranty. You might see the term 'warranted sound' or 'warranted in foal to a certain stallion', etc. A warranty is described under section 61 of the Sale of Goods Act as 'an agreement with reference to goods which are the subject of a contract of sale but collateral to the main purpose of such a contract the breach of which gives rise to a claim for damages but not a right to reject the goods and treat the contract as repudiated'.

What does this actually mean? All contracts are made up of terms, which can be conditions or warranties. They give rise to different remedies. A warranty is, if you like, a type of extra guarantee in addition to the terms and conditions of the contract. It can cover the horse generally – 'warranted in all respects' – or can be limited, or may be given in one particularly important aspect of the contract, e.g. – 'warranted proven brood mare'. It would be foolish as a seller to give a warranty for something you could not predict or had no control over, such as 'warranted sound for five years' or 'warranted to breed further foals'. Warranties only cover facts as at sale, for instance 'warranted sound' – as at this minute. Agents can give warranties but they should be very sure they are only giving warranties for things for which they have authority to do so.

If you buy at auction, you will see that some of the horses are 'warranted'. The auctioneers themselves will not give warranties. You will therefore usually hear an auctioneer use a phrase such as 'Seller warrants...' before the bidding starts. They are passing on what the seller has told them. Thus the auctioneer himself or his company would not be responsible if the horse failed to live up to its warranty. You would have to pursue the seller direct, unless for some reason the auctioneer was acting outside his authority and actually giving the warranty himself. The Sale of Goods Act does not apply to auction purchases.

If your contract or warranty has a time limit during which time you can return the horse for any reason or a specific reason as stated, then you must act within that period if you do want to return the horse or if the horse is not as stated in the contract. You will lose your right of automatic return of the horse under the condition if you don't keep within the time limit. This does not apply where there has been fraud. In all cases, warranty or not, inform the seller as soon as there is, or you think there might be, a problem. The problem must of course have arisen within a reasonable time after purchase. You cannot buy a horse and then when it contracts laminitis six years later, go back and complain to the seller. Some things will be difficult to detect immediately; for instance it may take time to reach the conclusion that a mare warranted as being in foal actually isn't.

If the horse dies or is badly injured after you have indicated you are returning it, then the seller may have to accept it, provided you as the buyer did not cause the death or injury in the first place.

Buying and selling horses can be a fraught business. The caring owner when selling will want to try and ensure that their horse goes to a caring and experienced home and will be well looked after. The ungenuine seller will be looking to offload a horse as quickly as possible, hoping that a problem does not show itself within too short a time. Buying a horse is a major purchase and is often the key to your future riding career. You may find it surprising that anyone can buy a horse at any time and in any circumstances without having to show that they are in any way suitable to have a horse or know anything about looking after it. One minute you can be having your second riding lesson in the protective confines of an indoor school with a qualified teacher, and the next you can be steering half a ton of unpredictable muscle with very little brain on a road through busy traffic – quite frightening when you think about it.

Insurance

The law does not as yet expect you to be licensed, qualified or otherwise regulated in order to buy a horse, but the one thing that cannot be emphasised too much is the need for at least third party liability insurance. This is insurance that will pay out compensation if somebody makes a claim against you for an accident or injury that may have been your fault, or the legal expenses involved in you either defending or settling a claim over a contract dispute; but do check the policy carefully.

It may be wise for you to consider taking out a separate legal expenses insurance policy which would enable you to make a claim with the legal expenses covered, although there does not appear to be a great market for this type of policy as yet. This is the sort of insurance that would allow you to make a claim against somebody else if you thought they were at fault and they had injured you or your horse, breached a contract, or damaged any property. You may never need to use it, but if you do it is something that you will be eternally thankful you have taken out. If you are a member of a body such as the Countryside Alliance, the British Horse Society (gold level and above), etc. you may find that you have insurance cover through them, but do check the nature of the cover carefully. You might find you are covered if you are a member of an affiliated riding club, otherwise look at your ordinary household build-ings and contents policy, which sometimes includes legal expenses.

None of these policies may cover a claim for veterinary negligence, but do check with the insurers.

Points to watch when buying

If you do get into a dispute over buying and selling a horse, then suc-cessfully making or defending a claim will depend not so much on who said what or what was written down but what are the real facts, how far these can be proved no matter what was said or written down, what can be proved to have been said and what was understood by what might or might not have been said. Documentary evidence is important, but not always conclusive.

When you are buying a horse it is prudent to ask as much as possible and even write down your question checklist beforehand, whereas in selling a horse it is probably prudent to stick to saying only factual points that cannot be misunderstood, unless you are absolutely confident that the horse will live up to your statements. The same goes for any written assurances you are asked to give.

As a buyer, once you accept that you will never buy the 100% perfect horse 100% of the time you are being realistic. Most sales and purchases of horses go through with no problems. Most sellers are honest and genuine people selling for a good reason or in the course of their business. Dealers do get a bad press, but the good ones will know that reputation is all and they will want repeat business. You can avoid problems to a large extent by considering the following points:

- Do your preparation and homework before buying. Don't be rushed into buying something you are not sure of. There *is* always another horse out there.

- Be realistic as to your ability and needs. If you overhorse yourself you will get problems, but they will not necessarily be the seller's fault.
- Do listen to your instincts.
- Don't pay out more than you could comfortably afford to write off if everything goes completely wrong. In particular, do not put yourself into debt unnecessarily to purchase a horse. Horses are worth what people will pay for them. If you have a nagging feeling that you are paying more for a horse than you either wanted to or you should be, then you probably are. If this doesn't matter to you, then go ahead and stop worrying. It's your money, you can do what you like with it. If it will worry you for years afterwards that you might have paid 'too much' for a horse, or you can't really afford it, then don't pay it. The horse that is right for you will be worth its price.
- Do be aware that any sort of litigation with what might be termed the 'average' horse can be uneconomic and sometimes you will have no other option than just to lose money and put it down to experience.
- Don't fall in love with a horse just because of its four white socks/long mane and tail/ability to eat a mint from its owner's mouth. Do try not to buy out of sympathy, unless you understand fully why you are buying the horse and you have the time and the facilities to sort it out. Equally, don't take on a horse such as a rehabilitated thoroughbred just because you think it will be a cheap way of getting a well-bred horse. It won't, and those who are involved in the rehabilitation and rehoming of rescued or problem animals are in the main extremely fussy about where they go.
- Buy as far as you can from someone with a reasonable and widespread reputation who has been in the business for a while and can offer such things as a money back or exchange scheme and a trial period, or if you are buying from a private individual buy from someone recommended. This will not always be possible and in practice most people rely for their purchases on advertisements in the many horse publications or in their local saddlery.
- Do try the horse as far as possible and get it vetted. This is an area of horse law where prevention is easily better than cure.

Chapter 7
Loaning Horses

Loaning horses, either having one on loan yourself or putting one out on loan, can be a satisfactory solution to a horse problem for two people. There are factors for and against loaning horses, whether you want one on loan yourself or want to put one out on loan.

If you are thinking of putting your horse out on loan do consider carefully whether it is the right arrangement for the horse. If the horse is very old and needs special care, or perhaps is quite young but with an injury which will rule out its being ridden or taking part in any activities for the rest of its life, then it may well be kinder to take the admittedly very difficult decision and have it put down. If on the other hand you have a pony which you've outgrown, but you want it back in the future for another member of the family, or you want to put it out on a short-term loan, perhaps because you are pregnant or at university, then it can be an ideal solution. If you take a horse on loan, then all you will avoid is the purchase price; after that it should be more or less as if the horse is your own, unless you have agreed differently with the owner.

Cost is a factor. If you buy a horse you will have to pay for it. If you loan a horse you usually avoid the purchase price but there may be a cost if it is actually being leased to you for a specific purpose. For instance, a stallion may be leased, or rented, for stud purposes for a period of time for a fee.

Ownership of a loan horse

Do not let anyone persuade you that a loan horse automatically becomes yours in certain circumstances – i.e. where the owner does not visit it for a year and a day; where you school it up to a certain standard; if you have it on loan for over three years, etc. You will never actually own a loan horse. No matter how long you have it, you cannot acquire ownership just by the length of time you have had the horse on loan. Ownership always remains with the person who loaned the horse to you. There is no scheme for adopting horses. This may not matter to you, but if you own a horse and spend your time schooling it and generally improving it, then you have the choice as to whether to keep it and reap the benefit of a well-schooled horse, or sell it, hopefully at a profit. If you loan a horse, you may well improve it beyond recognition during the period of your loan, but the owner can come and take it away at any time and there is no compensation for you for the hours of schooling or the strict feeding regime you have put in place. You may be someone who is quite happy to take on a horse on loan for the purpose of improvement as you enjoy the challenge, but this will frustrate others.

You can sell a horse of your own or put it on loan. You cannot sell a horse you have on loan or loan it to anybody else without the permission of the owner. The horse is not yours to sell or loan. It doesn't matter if you have had the horse for ten years without the owner coming anywhere near it, it is still not yours.

Theft and conversion

If you do sell it, it can be theft or an offence called 'conversion', or both. Theft is 'the dishonest appropriation of property belonging to another with the intention of permanently depriving the owner of that property' (Theft Act 1968, section 1.) Theft requires both a mental element to commit the offence as well as the actual act of the offence, in this case the dishonest taking of the horse or item. In legal terms these are called the *mens rea* (the mental element) and the *actus reus* (the physical act of carrying out the offence). You need to *intend* to take the horse and *permanently deprive* the owner of it and you need to actually *take* it. If either the mental or physical element, or part or parts of them are missing, there may not be a theft as per the legal definition. This would be the case, for instance, where someone borrowed a horse but always intended to return it, even if they were somehow prevented from doing so. There would be no intention to permanently deprive.

Conversion is where a thing, in this case a horse, is taken over and the rightful owner deprived of possession by someone else using it. The difference between theft and conversion is basically that in many cases, in conversion the horse or item will have been or is quite properly and legally in your possession to begin with, such as a horse on loan. You do not necessarily have to take it in the first place. At some point, though, you will form the intention to deal with the horse as if it were your own.

There is, however, such a thing as 'conversion by taking'. This is where someone takes a horse without the authority of the owner and with the intention of asserting a right over it. This would cover taking someone's horse and using it without their consent. You may actually intend to give it back, but you will have taken it without authority in the first place. It will not be theft as you do not intend to permanently deprive the owner of it.

It can also be conversion when you continue using a horse without permission where you may have had permission previously and the permission has been withdrawn, or where you refuse to give the horse back, say at the end of a loan period. It is a complicated area of law and if you suspect someone of either stealing or disposing of your horse while on loan, you will need to take legal advice as soon as possible.

As a matter of practicality, if you suspect theft or conversion you should alert the police as soon as possible, particularly if there is a local Horse Watch Scheme. Alert all local dealers, riding schools, livery yards, auctioneers, insurers, knacker's yards and the like – in fact, you can go as far as you like in circulating details of the missing horse. What you must not do, however, is advertise a reward for the return of the horse suggesting that if you get the horse back you will not make any enquiries as to how it disappeared or that there will be no prosecution for theft. If you have leaflets printed with this on, then even the printers can be liable! To do this is a criminal offence under the Theft Act 1968. Although you can do your best in alerting sale yards and auctioneers, what often happens is that an unscrupulous seller will take your horse to the sale but it will never get as far as the auction ring. It will be sold from the lorry or trailer in the car park, with no questions asked. It is essential therefore that you go yourself to as many sales or auctions as possible, to see if the horse is there. There is no doubt that this is a time-consuming, expensive and soul-destroying task.

Protective measures

Ensure that your horse is insured against theft. This is not automatically in every insurance policy. Conversion may not count as theft – again, check specifically with your insurers and if you put your horse on loan, notify them and send a copy of the loan agreement to them.

Freeze-marked horses are less likely to be taken or sold on and can be traced using freeze-mark companies. Some horses have numbers branded into their hooves. These will grow out in time if not replaced, but anyone wanting to steal or convert a horse will be less likely to want to risk having a horse around long enough for the feet to grow out to remove the numbers.

If your horse is loaned out, make sure you always keep its original papers and passport documents in a safe place away from where the horse is kept, together with identifying photographs and videos. It will be more difficult for someone to sell a horse without original papers, particularly where they are very important. This applies equally to your own horse, even when not on loan. Don't forget to update papers as your horse grows or changes colour, as many do particularly greys. Thieves can and do dye horses, but not usually the whole horse unless it is a particularly sophisticated crime. White socks or face markings can be altered.

You should also mark tack in an obvious way if that is loaned with the horse. Tack can have your postcode engraved on it, for instance; this is the method approved by the police, who suggest the postcode and the number of your premises or stables, or the first two digits if the number is long, or the first two letters of the name of the premises. Engrave on the stirrup bar and the underside of the saddle flap. Bridles are more difficult as they have a number of pieces, all of which will need to be engraved. Rugs too can be a problem. Thieves will go so far as to steal rugs off horses in the field, especially where it is isolated. You could for instance paint your postcode in large letters on the rugs, making them unattractive admittedly but also probably unsaleable and therefore not worth stealing.

The above all applies equally to horses and tack not out on loan.

Make sure your premises are secure and that any trailers kept on the premises are at least locked and at best locked away and disabled. Thieves will steal trailers and load stolen tack into them to transport it. Most tack thefts are thought to be targeted and premeditated.

Some insurance companies operate their own security methods and you should ask your insurers whether they have one.

Returning a loan horse

If you have a horse on loan, you can give it back if it is not suitable or it becomes impractical for you to keep a horse for some reason. If it is unsuitable then all you will have lost is your time and the cost of keeping the horse – which you would have incurred anyway if you had bought a horse – and possibly your nerve if the loan horse proves to have been loaned out because it is a problem animal. You will not have lost the purchase price or a large part of it, as you would if you had bought the horse, and will not have the problem or cost of trying to sell the horse. If the owner of your loan horse will not take it back or you cannot find the owner for some reason when you want to give the horse back, under the Tort (Interference with Goods) Act 1977 items can be sold when they don't belong to you as long as you comply with certain procedures. This includes horses, but as it is a complicated area of law you will need to consult a solicitor to check both that you will be able to sell and that the procedure is done correctly. If you have loaned out a horse you should have an agreement, of which more later in this chapter, which provides for the return of the horse and which can be enforced either through arbitration or mediation or by the court as a last resort.

If you buy a horse, it is more difficult to take it back if it is wrong as you will have to prove either that there has been a breach of contract entitling you to return the horse, or that you bought the horse due to a misrepresentation.

If you sell a horse, then it is usually gone and that is the last you see of it. This can sometimes be a good thing and a great relief, but it does mean that you have to trust that you have found your horse a good home where he or she will be well looked after. It is common to find owners trying to obtain news of horses they have sold even many years before.

Control over the horse

If you loan out a horse you can retain an element of control over its welfare and use. Do not, however, expect to loan out a horse and still dictate every move. The loanee (the person taking the horse on loan) will be entitled to something called 'quiet enjoyment' of the horse. This means that as long as the horse remains in their care in accordance with the conditions of the loan agreement, they are entitled to expect to be left alone to get on with it. There is some argument as to whether it is better to loan or share a horse and still keep it in your yard to keep an eye on it – or interfere, according to your view point – or whether it is better for a horse to go out of your orbit altogether. If the latter, you should still visit the horse from time to time to check on its welfare and the fact that it is still where it is supposed to be.

Sharing

Further options to loaning are sharing or part-ownership of a horse. The ownership of a shared horse will stay with the owner; all you will do is share the horse with the owner. You will not own all or any part of the horse at any time. Sharing arrangements can range from both parties, or indeed more than two parties, taking an equal share in the cost, care and riding of the horse, to the owner merely allowing you to ride out twice a week with no further input. The owner generally retains more control than if the horse is loaned out. Sharing can be quite frustrating if the owner always insists on taking precedence. A successful share arrangement largely depends on the parties getting on well, having the same outlook with regard to the horse and having a degree of flexibility. You should have a written agreement, as for a loan, and insurance, but no amount of writing will change a somewhat selfish person's attitude.

Part-ownership

Part-ownership means that you will be the owner of the horse to some degree. Racing or breeding syndicates such as those run by the National Stud or the Event Horse Owners Association often have very many 'owners' in part-ownership, with each owner 'owning' say a hundredth share of the horse, or rather more realistically, its value. You may part-own a horse with a successful rider where you are more interested in the training of the horse or in attending competitions where your horse is competing, but not so much bothered about, or even capable of, riding it.

Another common professional arrangement is for one person to own the horse completely, but for someone else to ride, compete on it or breed from it. Or you might have a half share with a friend; once again, ensure that the terms of the part ownership or the riding/competing/breeding arrangement are very clear, and have a proper written agreement. It is important to have a clear understanding of who is responsible for what, whether you half own an ageing Shetland pony or a good prospect in the Burghley horse trials. Think about the costs. Who decides when vets' bills are becoming uneconomic for a horse with a terminal lameness, where one party cannot bear to have it put down? If you pay all the entry fees for the horse to compete, are you entitled to keep all the winnings as well, or should the rider have them? Who owns the foal from a breeding arrangement? Questions such as these are in addition to the usual terms for the day-to-day responsibilities for the horse. The more professional the situation, and indeed it has to be said, the more money or prospective money involved, the more you should think about putting the arrangement on a proper business and commercial basis.

Bloodstock arrangements are a specialist area of law in themselves and beyond the scope of this book, but there are specialist niche solicitors who deal solely with anything to do with bloodstock and the racing industry.

Matching the horse and loanee

It is up to you to decide whether to loan or buy. Certainly there are more horses for sale than loan and many loan horses have either a particular problem or are perhaps elderly or only suitable for light work, so there may be some frustrating limitations on their use. But obtaining a horse whether by buying or loaning is a major step and getting the right horse will be crucial to the progress of your riding career.

In loaning horses you should take as much care as when buying, although you have to accept that a horse may be up for loan because it has some sort of imperfection. As long as this is acceptable to you, then fine. However, do be aware of two cases illustrating possible problems in loaning horses who may not be 100% reliable. First of all, the case of *Westphal and Barmer Ersatzkasse* v. *Alexander* (2000) (*Horse Law* (2000) Vol. 5, Iss. 6) suggests that if you put a horse out on loan to somebody, or indeed just lend it to them to ride or for a particular activity, then you do have a duty of care in law to make sure that the horse is suitable for that person. In this case, a horse was loaned to a friend of the owner. The friend was thrown and paralysed and sued the person who had loaned them the horse. The defendant, i.e. the person who had lent the horse to the friend, won the case on this occasion, but the judge pointed out that there was a duty of care, and that duty of care is that of the 'reasonable' owner or rider. Further, if the horse has any habits or quirks, such as for instance, spooking or bolting off, then the person loaning the horse must mention this. It may be that the person loaning the horse only suspects that this might happen even if it hasn't happened before; it should still be pointed out.

Fortunately, in this capacity the person loaning out the horse would not be expected to reach the standard of assessment of, say, a qualified riding instructor, but nevertheless the law will expect some sort of assessment to be carried out. This may not be the standard assessment expected of, say, a riding school, but certainly if you are loaning your horse out to someone or just letting them ride it as a favour, you should either know the person's riding ability well, or make sure that you see them ride the horse at all paces and handle him, both in a safe environment such as a school and on the road. Satisfy yourself that the loanee or rider will be able to cope with your horse. Of course, if the rider gives you totally misleading information about their ability or experience which is not apparent on an assessment, then you may not be at fault if anything happens, or at the very least the loanee, if an accident occurred, would be at least partially responsible for the consequences.

There would be a danger in taking this too far. For instance, what about relay races in gymkhanas, where four riders use the same pony? Is it realistic to suggest that between each heat every rider should have ten minutes' assessment on the pony to make sure that they are able to cope with it at walk, trot and canter? What about a situation where you and a friend swap horses for a change? Say your horse and your friend love hunting but you don't? It would be a pity if this point were allowed to go too far, thus limiting people to riding their own horses, but if you are thinking of loaning out a horse or letting someone ride your horse, then do try to satisfy yourself that they appear reasonably competent and have the ability that they claim. You could ask for references on this point, or you may be entitled to go by the loanee's qualifications if, for instance, they are a BHSAI (see Chapter 2) or have some sort of equine riding degree, or even just by the fact that they have had their own horse for a number of years but for some reason now need to take one on loan. In those cases it would probably be safe for you to assume that they do have a certain level of ability.

It would probably be wise to be cautious about loaning your horse to a complete novice, not only from the practical aspect of ensuring that your horse is well looked after, but also from a possible legal point shown in the case of *Flack* v. *Hudson* (2000) (*The Times*, 6 November). Mrs Sherry Flack was riding a horse with the consent of its owner when the horse shied at a tractor. The horse bolted and sadly Mrs Flack fell and died from head injuries. Her husband sued the owner and the tractor driver, but the tractor driver was later found to be not at fault at all. Neither was it found that Mrs Flack was in any way to blame for her own accident. She apparently had some riding experience but could not be said to be an experienced rider.

Mr Flack, the widower, brought his case under section 2(2) of the Animals Act 1971. The plaintiff (now called the claimant) said that the horse that Mrs Flack had been riding was extremely unsafe in traffic. It was argued that this was a specific problem of this horse and that Mrs Flack had not been told about it. There seems to have been some difference of opinion in the evidence in that Mrs Hudson, who was the person being sued, either denied that the horse was traffic shy or alternatively argued that she had told Mrs Flack of this problem. It seems that Mrs Hudson's husband had been injured by the horse previously when it had bolted in similar circumstances. Eventually it was found that Mrs Hudson was liable for the accident.

If you take a horse on loan from somewhere such as the International League of Protection for Horses, or any of the other animal welfare societies, you can expect to be closely vetted before being matched with a horse and to be refused if they do not think you suitable. If you are accepted as a suitable loanee, then you can expect to be closely monitored after you take possession of the horse, with officers of the charity retaining the right to inspect the horse and the premises where it is kept at any time. It is however likely that if you have a horse on loan from one of the charities for a long period, the inspections may become less frequent; they will not however cease altogether. The charity will retain the right to take the horse back at any time.

Loan agreements

Loans can be permanent or for a fixed period, or open to renewal on a periodic basis, or even for a specific purpose, however long that takes, e.g. to breed a foal, or to qualify a horse for Wembley, or to break a youngster and bring it on to affiliated level dressage. If there are limits to the extent of the loan either in time or purpose, then this should be made very clear in the loan agreement.

It is strongly advised that you always have a written loan agreement. The point about such an agreement is not that it will protect you in all circumstances, because it won't – as in buying and selling horses, if someone is specifically out to defraud you, then it is likely that they will do so and you will be unlikely to be able to protect yourself 100%. What the loan agreement will do, however, is prove that there was a loan in the first place, thus sidestepping the problem of someone maintaining that the horse was given to them as a gift. But do ensure that *no money* changes hands on a loan. If a dispute arose, a payment, however small, could be alleged to be a sale or purchase price, thus showing that there was not a loan, it was a sale or purchase.

The loan agreement will also set out the terms and conditions of the loan and what each party understands by them. The important point about the loan agreement is that it makes both parties think very carefully about what they are entering into prior to doing so, and consider in detail what they each want from the arrangement. The British Horse Society and the Country Land and Business Association both draft loan agreements – the BHS's can be viewed on its website. There is also a sample loan agreement in Appendix 1 of this book. Bear in mind that in an agreement you are unlikely to cover every eventuality but there are a few basics that should always be covered.

You can attempt to put anything you like in a loan agreement and the details can be as brief or as detailed as you like. For instance, you could just use one line – 'The horse should be adequately cared for in respect of feed, water, stabling, grazing, tack, shoeing, worming and general welfare' – or you could state precisely what you want, – e.g. 'The horse shall be shod every eight weeks at least using the services of...', 'The horse shall be wormed every six to eight weeks using...' [whatever particular preparations you want]'. The problem with including such detail is the difficulty in enforcing it. How are you going to know, unless you turn up every six to eight weeks with the wormer, that this requirement is being fulfilled? Does it really matter as long as the horse is wormed and remains in good health? You may have a great deal of faith in your present farrier, but there are other good ones around who will shoe your horse just as well. If you make your agreement too detailed and specific, you run the risk of potential loanees thinking the loan is not worth the bother.

Your loan agreement should at least state the following.

Loan only

That it is an agreement for a loan and not a sale, that ownership has not passed and will not pass under any circumstances and that the horse must not be sold, loaned out or hired out, etc without the owner's express written permission and full knowledge.

Description of horse, tack and equipment

There should be a description of the horse including colour, injuries, any freeze marks, scars, allergies, vices, habits, etc. You could do this in a separate schedule attached to the loan agreement and you could even include a photograph of the horse taken from different angles.

You should do the same with any tack and equipment sent with the horse. You should make provision for replacement of tack but you must accept that there will be a certain amount of normal wear and tear.

Consider having the horse vetted as you would when buying a horse (see Chapter 4). This shows to both loaner and loanee any defects the horse has. It will also provide an objective view and evidence of the horse's state of health at the commencement of the loan. It might prevent a loanee trying to say that a horse had a particular problem or injury before it was loaned, when in reality it has arisen since the start of the loan. If the owner appears somewhat reluctant to have this done, perhaps the prospective loanee should wonder why. It may be best to choose an independent vet. If there are any specific problems outside the normal vetting procedure either party wants checking, make sure the vet knows beforehand so he or she can bring the correct equipment, i.e. x-ray machines.

Period of loan

You should set out the period of the loan, Do you want an option to renew on the same terms at the end, or renegotiate?

Notice period

There should be a period of notice for either side to end the agreement and you should state whether this can be orally or in writing. You should include provision for immediate termination of the loan if there is any major breach of the agreement or if there is, for instance, any evidence of cruelty or mistreatment towards the horse.

Where horse is kept

It should be stated where the horse is to be kept and how. You should include provision for the loanee to notify you should they wish to move the horse for any reason, and for you to be entitled to refuse to give that permission and have the horse returned.

Payment of expenses

You should set out very carefully who does what and who pays for it. For instance, who pays for the feed, shoes, transport, vaccinations, vet's fees, insurance, entry fees to competitions, etc. If you are a loanee, be very careful about giving an open-ended agreement that you will be responsible for vet's fees to an uncapped limit. You want to avoid being left with a horse that it would be economic to have put down, but the owner is insisting that you carry on paying vet's fees even where this may be pointless. This is particularly important when you take on a horse with a known injury or health problem. There may be an exclusion on any insurance policy for a known problem, therefore vet's fees will not be covered. Do you perhaps want to try to get the owner to pay for any vet's fees connected with the existing problem, while you pay for anything else? Of course you could give notice to return the horse if you find yourself having to pay continual and excessive vet's fees, but you may find yourself still looking after the horse for another month, three months or whatever your agreement is. You could perhaps say that you will be responsible generally for vet's fees up to a certain amount for a known problem or only as far as any insurance allows for other things, and after that it will be the owner's responsibility. This might stop an unscrupulous owner refusing to take the horse back and wanting you as the loanee to keep it going. There is nothing wrong with loaning out a horse with a known problem as long as the loanee is made fully aware of the extent of the problem and the problem is not one that might be dangerous – a horse that has sudden fits, for instance. If neither of you want the responsibility for possibly long-term vet's bills, then there may be only one alternative and that is to have the horse put down.

The owner might want to argue that they have been straight with you about the horse's problems, if you later quibble over vet's bills, and you will have to take it as you find it. If the horse is an absolute gem in many ways, then you may find the payment of vet's fees a small price to pay.

Insurance

If you are the person taking the horse on loan you may want to make sure that it is insured at all times by paying the insurance premium yourself. It may be worth it for peace of mind. In any case, if a horse is on loan, the insurers must be informed and usually you will find that they want a copy of the loan agreement.

If as the owner you are paying for the insurance the loanee should be given a copy of the insurance certificate and a term put in the agreement that the policy must be complied with. You may find that if the policy is not complied with it becomes invalid, and if either you or the loanee then make a claim it may not be met. There can be problems with this. For instance, there may be a time limit for notifying the insurance company of a potential claim. If you are insuring the horse yourself but you don't see it very often, then if the loanee doesn't advise you of a potential problem you may find that the time limit has passed for making a claim.

The loanee should ensure that they can comply with the terms of the insurance. For instance, are they at a livery yard where the tack is kept in, say, an insecure redundant caravan, but the policy requires it to be kept in a securely locked brick-built building with alarms? There may be little either you or the loanee can do to change this situation and you may have to insist that the loanee takes the tack home every night and that it is covered under their household policy. If it is just a matter of putting a simple lock on a door, it might be worth paying for this to be done yourself.

You should also make sure that any payments made under the policy are made to the person to whom they are due, i.e. the person who may already have paid vet's fees or suffered any other loss. You don't want, as the owner, to pay the vet's fees as you go along and then to find that the insurance policy issues a cheque in the name of the loanee who then refuses to reimburse you. There are remedies for this, but there are equally more practical solutions that you can take to stop it arising in the first place. Cheques should, however, always be issued in the policy-holder's name.

Authority of loanee

You should make clear the extent of the authority of the loanee with regard to veterinary attention and in particular when the horse can be put down. Clearly if there was an emergency situation with the vet standing by to put the horse down, you would not want the loanee frantically trying to telephone you to comply with the agreement to obtain your consent, but your mobile phone is switched off. You may want to insert a clause that as long as the horse is being put down under veterinary advice and recommendation, then the loanee can go ahead. In non-emergency situations you may want to be informed if at all prac-tical. This is one of the areas where there would have to be a certain degree of trust between the parties that the horse's welfare would be the main concern.

Purpose of loan

You should set out the purpose of the loan – breaking, schooling, general riding, etc. Is there anything that the horse cannot do or that you as the owner do not want him to do, e.g. cross-country or hunting? Is there any equipment that must not be used, e.g. severe bits, spurs, balancing reins, etc? If the loan has a specific purpose, then the loanee will want to make it clear that they will not be in breach of the agreement just because that specific purpose has not been fulfilled, such as schooling a horse to novice dressage standard. There may be all sorts of reasons why the purpose has not been achieved – the horse is not up to it, it has been lame, etc. The converse of this is that the owner may want to take the horse back if it is clear it is not doing as well as expected with the loanee.

Riding the horse

Set out who can and cannot ride the horse, or state that it is to be left to the loanee's discretion. It is probably unreasonable to be too restrictive over this, unless you know the horse is a difficult or sensitive ride and should, for instance, only be ridden by those with considerable experience. It would also not be fair to expect to retain a specific right for you or your family to ride the horse when it is out on loan, say in the school holidays or whatever. If you have a good relationship with your loanee, no doubt there would be no problem with you riding the horse from time to time – perhaps when you visit – but to expect the loanee to do all the work and you to ride the horse would probably be unacceptable.

At loanee's risk

If you are loaning out a horse, put in a clause that states that the loanee has had an opportunity to inspect and try the horse before taking it on, and that all the horse's faults and vices have been disclosed prior to loan. Make sure that this actually happens. You should then say that the loanee understands that this having been done, they are taking the horse at their own risk. It may not protect you completely if something happens due to your negligence or because of something you have failed to disclose, but it will help if there is an accident. You cannot, in any agreement or contract, exclude your own liability for personal injury or death where that has occurred because of your negligence.

Authority over horse

You should make provision for inspecting and visiting the horse from time to time if you are loaning it out; but on the other hand the loanee should have a provision for something called 'quiet enjoyment'. This means that, basically, having made all the arrangements and the horse having been handed over, the loanee will be left alone to get on with the horse as if he or she owned the horse, unless both the person loaning the horse and the loanee want to have a particularly close relationship with frequent contact. A loanee would almost certainly find it unacceptable to be expected to be responsible for the horse both practically and financially, but the person loaning out the horse wanted to retain a large degree of control, in particular retaining the right to ride the horse at will. If this is the situation, then a sharing agreement may be more suitable than a loan.

Future sale of the horse

Do you want to put in a clause giving the loanee first option to buy the horse if you do decide to sell? If so, do you want to state the price now, which might work in the loanee's favour, or make provision for how the price is going to be decided later, i.e. by asking a reputable dealer what the market price for the horse would be at the time of sale? This might favour the seller, perhaps because the horse has been vastly improved while out on loan. But would the loanee want to pay a higher price when it is he or she who has made the improvement? Is it fair to expect them to?

Arbitration

You should put in an arbitration clause. This means that if there is a dispute, then instead of immediately terminating the loan, which may be in neither person's best interest, or rushing off to law, which may be costly and uneconomic, the matter is referred to, say, an independent vet or a Fellow of the British Horse Society for determination. The clause should say that all parties involved will abide by that person's decision. *But note –* you may be prevented from taking an action to court if there is an arbitration clause in the agreement.

   You should get the nominated person's agreement to act before putting it in the agreement. You should make provision for both parties to bear the cost of the arbitrator's fees equally, but any other fees involved should be borne by the party incurring them. If you agree to share all costs equally, you might find yourself bearing half of a very expensive lawyer's bill where the other party has taken legal advice.

Welfare society agreements

Bodies such as the International League of Protection for Horses will have their own loan agreements and you will be unlikely to be able to change these substantially. If you would feel uncomfortable being closely monitored, then you should probably not ask for a horse from a welfare society.

Sharing or leasing agreements

Agreements for sharing or leasing horses follow much the same pattern as a loan agreement, except where the agreement is of a more commercial nature, in which case you may want to engage the services of a blood stock agent or a blood stock solicitor. This could be the case with, say, a stallion leasing agreement.

Selling the horse

If you make your arrangements too detailed, you may find difficulty in loaning your horse at all. There does have to be a certain degree of respect and trust between the parties and again you may find that instinct is a good guide. Certainly as an owner make sure you keep an eye on your horse from time to time, and as a loanee perhaps you should be wary of an owner who doesn't appear to care what happens to their horse. Although, as previously mentioned, you cannot acquire a horse merely by passage of time, if the owner does not appear to be interested in the horse at all then you could offer to buy it after a while if you feel that you want to keep the horse permanently. There is no obligation on the owner to sell to you and also no obligation to sell to you at a low price because you have been loaning the horse. If you have the money and you feel strongly enough, then even if you feel the price being asked is too much you may want to go ahead and buy the horse. If on the other hand the price is a matter of concern to you, just carry on with the loan for as long as possible. You have to remember though that it is a loan and that the horse can go back at almost any time if the owner wishes.

As an owner, if you think that you will not be bothered about the horse long-term and in particular you feel that there are no circumstances in which you want the horse back, then you may as well sell and be done with it. That way at least you have a capital sum, perhaps to buy another horse, and you do not have the constant worry of checking up on the horse and wondering what you would do if the loanee decided to return it to you.

Companion horses

Do be wary of advertisements looking for companion horses. Again, these can be genuine, but there has been publicity about people who have sent their horses off as a companion horse, only to find that when they go to check on them or perhaps take them back again, the horse is not available or has disappeared. The people who place these advertisements can be very plausible. They will take you to very nice accommodation and show you the youngsters for whom your horse will be a companion, and for a short time after the agreement they will send you photographs of your horse looking apparently well and happy. You may then find that contact tails off, or you will get a telephone call or a letter telling you that unfortunately your horse had to be put down due to illness or injury, or even that it has died. Or you may not hear anything at all and if you do go to see your horse in his 'companion home', there will be nothing there or no-one who has heard of your horse or the people to whom you loaned him.

These people will have sold the horse on, either for meat or for riding, probably to equally innocent purchasers. If your horse really is only suitable as a companion, then unless you can guarantee his home, you may well want to consider for your own peace of mind and for the sake of your horse's welfare, putting the horse down. This may be a better option than an uncertain and perhaps unhappy future. You could also see whether one of the horse welfare charities would take the horse in retirement.

If you do get caught out in the way described above, you could of course always try and have the person prosecuted for theft or conversion, or sue them for the value of the animal; but this is likely to be a long and drawn out business, not easy to prove and uneconomic. You will also have the problem of locating the perpetrators in the first place. Prevention in these cases is certainly better than trying to effect a cure.

From all that has been said in this chapter, don't think loaning is just a big potential problem. When it works well, it offers a real solution to a possible problem and makes two people and a horse very happy.

Chapter 8

Keeping a Horse at Home or at Livery

There are two main options on where to keep your horse: at home using your own land and stabling, or at livery or on someone else's land.

Keeping the horse at livery basically means that you keep your horse at someone else's premises in return for a fee. What you get for your money will very much depend on the individual agreement you have with the livery yard, and on the facilities available.

If you do have a choice of livery yards within your area it is recommended that you visit them to see which one would be best for your needs. You may find as a novice rider that you would feel intimidated with a horse at livery in a professional yard; if you are very experienced and do a lot of competing, on the other hand, you will need to look for a livery yard that can offer facilities such as an indoor school, availability of jumping facilities, space for a trailer or horsebox if you can't keep it at home, and access to good riding.

Many areas will have a very restricted choice of livery and if you do not have the option of keeping your horse at home or purchasing property that would enable you do so, then you may just have to make the best of it. Having said that, the atmosphere, facilities and management of a livery yard are very important to the enjoyment of your horse and if the only options are livery yards that you are not keen on, perhaps it might be best to delay the purchase of a horse until you can keep it at home or until you move to an area with more choice of yards.

There are advantages and disadvantages to both options of where to keep your horse. If you keep it at home it is under your own supervision all the time, it is easily accessible, you can look after it in your own individual way and, for example, nobody else will be using the wheelbarrows just when you want them. On the other hand, livery yards do offer some company, somebody else to hack out with or to help you with your schooling, and there may be somebody available to look after your horse if you are ill or go away on holiday. One compromise could be that you either use your own land or purchase a property with stabling and grazing and use part of it for your own horse and let out some of it for another livery or liveries yourself.

This is an option that could work well if you get the right person but could prove a disaster if you don't.

Even if you have only one other person, you might want to draw up a proper livery contract and it is recommended that you take out at least third party insurance. You might also want to check that you are not going to be classified as a business and subject to rates, etc.

Livery yards

Unlike riding establishments, livery yards do not need a licence to operate, and there isn't one coherent set of laws that applies to livery yards. If the yard is mixed – part riding school or trekking centre, part livery – then the Riding Establishments Act will apply to the riding part but not the livery part. Livery yard owners do not need any particular qualifications or training to own or run a livery yard. There is no definition of a livery yard and you will find great variation in what is on offer.

Livery yards are, however, subject to the general law where it applies. For instance, if there was a fire, and damage, injury or even death was caused as a result of the yard having no proper fire precautions to deal with it, then the yard would be likely to be liable under the general law of negligence if nothing else. It would not be a defence to say that the requirements under the Riding Establishments Act do not apply and therefore there was no need for fire precautions. A responsible livery yard owner should try and comply with the requirements of the Riding School Licence as far as possible – see Chapter 1. The yard will require public liability insurance.

It is perhaps arguable that there should be standards set for livery yards just as much as for riding establishments, but the argument against this is that many livery yards run very successfully with conscientious owners even without being required officially to adhere to certain standards. If there is too much 'red tape' attached to running a livery yard, then many people may not bother to offer such facilities, thus restricting availability. There is a list of British Horse Society approved livery yards, which are required to meet certain standards, and you may find that the livery yard you are contemplating is also a riding school and therefore will need to be licensed and will be subject to inspections.

There are a number of different types of livery and it may be possible to choose the type most suited to you and your horse, although not all livery yards will offer a choice. The main possible options are described here.

Grass livery or grazing only

This is where the horse is just turned out for grazing and a stable is not provided, although a field shelter or a shed might be. Depending on your agreement, you might also be allowed to use general facilities that exist, such as an arena, and of course you should be entitled to use the electricity and water if available. Even though your horse will be kept out or at grass under this type of livery, you can probably arrange for it either to be do-it-yourself, whereby you are responsible for the supervision of your horse, any extra feeding, rugging up and clearing the field, etc., or for these services to be provided by the yard owners or managers, possibly at extra cost.

If you just rent a field, rather than have grass livery within a mixed yard, you – and almost certainly the person renting to you – will want a written agreement which could amount to a more formal rental agreement or lease. This can be drafted to include various conditions as to who is responsible for what – fencing, upkeep, fertilising, etc. – and what can and can't be done – placing jumps on the land, adding extra horses and the like.

Usually, once you have rented the land you can treat it as your own as long as you stick to the terms of any agreement, and if you do the landlord should leave you alone to get on with it. The land should be put in a safe and secure condition by the landlord before renting it out, unless the landlord agrees with the proposed tenant that they will put it in good repair. If this is the agreement, then both sides should be very clear about what is to be done and to what standard.

Occupying land in this way can amount to a formal tenancy and may require proper eviction proceedings before a tenant can be removed.

Do-it-yourself livery

Do-it-yourself livery is probably the most popular type of livery and is just what it says: you will pay the yard owners or managers a weekly or monthly fee and in return you will be allowed to use certain facilities to look after your horse yourself. It is probably the most popular type of livery. When we speak of do-it-yourself livery, it is usually taken to mean that a stable and some form of grazing or turnout are provided. The extent of the grazing and turnout will depend on the extent of the land available and the number of horses that need to use it. General upkeep and maintenance of the facilities will usually be the responsibility of the managers or the owners of the yard, although of course you will be required to use the facilities properly and keep them in good order as far as possible.

The actual horse and the care of it will be the owner's responsibility. The livery yard owners will be unlikely to do anything towards the care of the horse unless specifically agreed. Some do-it-yourself yards will, for instance, put feed and hay over the door of the horse's stable in the morning, or perhaps bring it in in the evening, but there is likely to be an extra charge for this.

Do-it-yourself livery can be as basic as a home-built stable with a small turnout yard and a hosepipe for filling buckets, or it can be as grand as large purpose-built loose boxes, acres of grazing, indoor and outdoor schools, cross-country courses and 24-hour surveillance cameras.

If you are a livery yard owner, what you are doing is granting some-body – the 'licensee' – a 'licence' to use certain buildings and facilities. This means that you are really just 'allowing' them to use certain facilities. The 'licence' can be relatively easily withdrawn, usually by giving notice to the licensee. The notice period should be in your livery contract and is usually 28 days. You should make sure that you have a properly drafted agreement to ensure that both parties are very clear on what the livery fee covers. You should be careful that you are not granting a full tenancy to the occupier of a stable, although this would be very unusual. To guard against this you should have a clause in your livery agreement that entitles you to move horses around to different stables at any time and makes it clear that no livery has the sole right to any particular stable. You may not need to move horses, but you should retain the right to do so.

Part livery

Part livery is where livery facilities are provided and in the main the owner of the horse will be responsible for the horse's welfare and care, but part of the work will be undertaken by the yard owners or staff. For instance, if you have to be at work very early each day, your agreement may say that the yard will be responsible for all the morning work to do with the horse, whereas you take over to do evening stables and riding.

Full livery

When you put your horse at full livery, all facilities and care are provided by the owners or managers of the yard and all you have to do is ride. Even that can sometimes be handed over too, and all you then have to do is the patting. Full livery can be a good arrangement for those with demanding jobs or who are away a lot but still want to ride, but it is of course the most expensive option. There should still be the usual agreement drawn up and insurance taken out. The insurance, with all liveries, should cover anyone who handles the horse whether or not they are employed by the yard. It is also possible to take out something called 'care, custody and control' insurance which should cover death or injury to the horses. Third party insurance may only cover people. In Appendix 2 of this book there is an example of a livery agreement which can be modified for part or do-it yourself livery, but do remember this is only an example. Your own agreement should reflect your own circumstances.

Working livery

Working livery should only be offered at licensed riding establishments. With this arrangement you agree with the riding school owner that the horse can be used to a certain extent in the riding school. Depending on the arrangement, you will either still remain responsible for the horse's care and welfare, or the riding school owner may be prepared to be responsible for part of its care in return for you as the owner allowing it to be used for lessons. This may result in a lower livery fee.

The riding school owner should ensure that the horse is fully insured for use as a school horse, both for injury to the horse and rider and third party injuries or accidents.

Again, there are pros and cons about the arrangement. If you have a horse that can take or needs a lot of work, then regular use in the school may be a good thing. You should, however, be very clear on the extent of the use of the horse as you do not want the horse being overworked to the point where you feel you cannot ride it, nor do you want it used at times when you might want to ride. You may find that the greatest demand for your horse is at weekends when many people have riding lessons and this may be the time when you yourself want to ride, so it may not necessarily be an ideal arrangement. You may also be unhappy about the level of rider that your horse is being used for and so you do need to discuss the arrangements very carefully with the riding school owner and get a very clear working livery agreement.

Livery agreements

In a livery agreement, consider the following points.

As a livery yard owner

- Make sure you set the basic weekly or monthly livery charge at a figure that covers all extras such as electricity, water, rates, insurance costs, maintenance, etc. You can make provision for a basic charge with extras added, e.g. an extra charge for parking of a trailer or horse box, or for use of indoor school or lights. You might find, however, that most people prefer one all-inclusive payment per week or month. Consider whether you need to charge VAT.

- Make it clear in your agreement exactly what the cost covers and make provision for increases if you wish. You could say that the cost will rise by the rate of inflation once every 12 months, or perhaps that it will increase from time to time but with, say, one month's notice to all parties in case someone does not want to pay the increased cost and chooses to move elsewhere.
- Have the fee payable in advance. Consider taking a deposit, returnable when the livery leaves only if everything is in order and there are no outstanding debts. You cannot sell the livery's horse to pay for any monies owing to you as the livery yard owner, unless there is provision for it in the livery contract. Even if there is, you may have to go through a series of specific procedures before you can do this. If it occurs, take proper legal advice before you do anything. The problem should only arise if the livery owner has disappeared, as otherwise you should have provisions in your contract to help you deal with such difficulties.
- Do address any problem of debt at an early stage, while the debt can still be recovered from the amount held on deposit, warning the owner that you may have to give notice if it happens again. Be sensitive however – there are cases of genuine hardship which perhaps deserve sympathy and some help if you afford it.
- Do not as the yard owner or manager pay the farrier, vet or for wormers, etc. for the livery. Insist that the money is either left out or given to you beforehand. No money, no shoes!

As a livery

- Will hay, straw and feed be provided by the livery yard owners and at what cost, or are liveries able to buy in their own? Is there a particular regime, for instance are all horses required to be on straw because this makes it easier to dispose of manure heaps, or are all horses required to be kept on a dust-free bedding which may be more expensive?
- If you are on part or full livery, is there a choice of feed or will your horse just be given what everyone else's gets? If you do choose something different and supply it yourself, will there be a reduction in cost?
- Will you be allowed to use your own vets and farriers, or will you be restricted to ones nominated by the yard?
- Does the yard have a standard worming regime or are you expected to worm your own horse regularly when required? Does the livery yard

owner check whether horses are properly wormed and inoculated and generally kept in good health?

- Does the livery yard owner reserve the right to call out a veterinary surgeon or a farrier if needed? This could cover the obvious such as when a horse has colic or has lost a shoe, but supposing the livery yard owner, or indeed the other liveries, call out a vet because they think a horse is not being looked after properly. Do they have the right to do this? Who would be responsible for costs in those circumstances? Would the yard owner want a provision in the agreement for a deposit, with the right to take such costs out of that, even though this may lead to bad feeling?
- Are there any restrictions on times you can be at the livery yard? If you have to be at work at 7.30AM there is no point in using a livery yard where you can't go in to look after your horse until 8AM; similarly, if you are supposed to be off the yard by 6PM and this may not only cause you problems getting home from work in time but also would restrict your ability to ride in the evenings, then don't go to that yard.
- Who is responsible for security? Is the yard going to be responsible if tack, trailers or horses are damaged or stolen, or do these remain the responsibility of the livery come what may, even where security is poor and an incident is the yard's fault? As always, do make sure that you have insurance and that the conditions of the insurance can be adhered to by the facilities at the yard. If they cannot, then your insurance may be invalid anyway. Does the yard have insurance against any claims made against it?
- What responsibilities will the livery yard owner take for accidents on the yard? Say, for instance, the owner allows a horse to be kept at livery on the yard when it is known to be dangerous and it will attack anyone who goes into its box. Clearly the answer is not to take on such horses in the first place, or if a horse does become dangerous in any way to make provision for notice to be given to the owner, but this may not always happen. The livery yard owner may never come down to the yard and may not be aware of the problem.

Division of responsibilities at livery

There is some debate over how far a livery yard owner's responsibilities extend and it may be a question of the degree of hands-on responsibility they have. Obviously with full and part livery the person looking after the horse under the agreement will be responsible for the horse to the extent that they are required to look after it. If the rider or the horse are injured as a result of something which is the responsibility of the livery yard owner, then the yard owner is likely to be liable. For instance, if they are responsible for maintenance of the fences between paddocks, but this is not done and horses are able to escape into other fields, perhaps kicking other horses, then the livery yard owner may well be responsible for the extent of the damage and for compensation. If on the other hand you as the rider put your horse out but then forget to close the gate properly and the horse escapes, then you would be responsible. The yard may not be responsible for damage caused in the course of normal 'horseplay' to your horse by other horses with which it is turned out, where there is no indication that any of the horses were known to be particularly aggressive.

The situation can be more difficult where yard owners or members feel that a horse is being neglected. Obviously there are times when a horse is neglected not necessarily through cruelty, but perhaps through ignorance. In some cases, the other owners can lead by example and hope that the owner concerned will follow suit. A responsible livery yard owner may want a quiet word with an owner who might not be looking after their horse properly, recognising that this may lead to the owner going elsewhere – but that may be no bad thing except that it may not improve the lot of the horse. There is an offence under the Protection of Livestock Act 1911 of, briefly, failing to take action to prevent unnecessary suffering, so do be careful of this. As a final sanction notice can be given to the owner, although if the aim is to improve the horse's situation this may not have the desired effect. All it might do is lead the owner to take the problem to another livery yard.

With working livery, as mentioned earlier, do make sure that all parties are very clear about what the horse can and cannot be used for, and make sure it is not overworked.

Planning permission

If you are thinking of starting up a livery stable or riding establishment, or of keeping your horse at home, you may need planning permission either to build new stables or use existing stables for the purpose of keeping a horse or horses. Planning permissions are a wide subject and it is not the intention of this book to go into it in great detail. Basic advice has to be that if you are buying a property to keep horses on, then check during the purchasing process that existing buildings used as stables have planning permission, or that planning permission will be given to erect stables or change the use of outbuildings to stables. If you are planning any construction connected with horses, do check with your local planning authority before you start as to whether planning permission will be necessary and if it is, what the conditions will be.

You will find that you usually need planning permission not only for stables but also for things like indoor schools, outdoor arenas, particularly if floodlit, and even horse walkers. You may not need planning permission if you are merely replacing something with a similar structure, e.g. replacing six dilapidated boxes with six new ones. If the necessary planning permission is not in existence, or you go ahead and build something and then find that planning permission was needed, the local authority can order those buildings to stop being used for horses, or even to be demolished, which is a waste of everybody's time and money. Retrospective planning permission can be granted, but this cannot be guaranteed.

If you are a tenant, or are considering renting land or buildings for equestrian purposes, you will not only have to check that basic planning permission is in order, but also that any tenancy or leasing agreement allows you to keep horses and/or carry on a business if that is what you intend to do. If you own the property, with or without a mortgage, you should check that there is no restriction on the keeping of animals or running of a business from that particular property, not only in your property deeds but also in your mortgage conditions.

In keeping your horse at home, you will not need planning permission for a stable or stables where they can be built within what is known as the 'curtilage' of a 'dwelling house'. 'Curtilage' is the legal term used generally speaking to mean 'garden'. There is no hard and fast rule on how big the garden has to be to come within the definition of curtilage. It may be that if you have a very big house, then the three acres or so surrounding it will still constitute a garden.

There will be limits on how big the stables can be and where in the garden they can be located, and these will be set out in a Town and Country Planning General Permitted Development Order, which may be changed from time to time. For instance, you may not be allowed to build a stable that is higher than the original house or that projects out from the front of a house where the house sits on a road. Realistically, the smaller the curtilage, the smaller the stable development might have to be.

Planning permission is not generally required for development for agricultural purposes, but horses are not generally regarded as agricultural animals and therefore planning permission may well be required.

If you have agricultural land and you want to graze a horse on it, then you will probably not need planning permission. However, the test is whether the land is solely grazing land. The land must be used totally or predominantly for grazing if planning permission is not to be required. You may get a situation where you have what is technically a field, that is a space enclosed by hedges or fencing, but there is no or very little grazing on it and the horse has to be fed in other ways, i.e. by the provision of regular hay and hard feed. The horse may well be kept in a shelter on that land. It could be said therefore that the predominant use of the land was for keeping the horse on rather than for grazing and therefore planning permission may be required.

You may get a situation where your land has mixed use. It may be the case that the fields are used for grazing horses, but you might also have put up a cross-country course using part of the hedging and part of the field, or erected permanent show jumps in the field. Putting up such jumps would amount to a change of use of the grazing land and so planning permission would be needed. Again, it would be a question of what is the predominant use of the land, which can be a very subjective view. If the jumps are used regularly, either by yourself or by liveries, then the jumping course may well be the predominant use. If on the other hand you keep your horse at home and you have put in one solid wooden fence to jump your horse over from time to time, then the grazing may still be the predominant use.

Field shelters may also require planning permission. A fixed shelter probably will require planning permission but if it is moveable then it may not. Again, there is a certain element of subjectivity. If there is a query and you are subject to an inspection by the local planning authority, to escape liability you should be able to show evidence of the shelter having been moved, i.e. that it is light enough to drag or that it has wheels so that it is mobile. Can you point to discoloured areas of grass where the shelter has stood for a period, then been moved to a different part of the field?

Planning permission may not be needed if it falls within a 'permitted development' but this generally only covers agricultural uses and property operated as a trade or business over a certain size. Talk things over with your local planning authority if in any doubt. If you do not want to alert the authority to any proposed developments, there are freelance planning consultants who can assist but there will be a fee.

Nuisance

You will not be allowed to keep horses or obtain planning permission for doing so where the keeping of them is likely to cause a nuisance in legal terms. This nuisance may not necessarily be because the horse itself is a nuisance, but you may find that you are not allowed to keep a manure heap, or you can only have a manure heap in a certain location or up to a certain size, as otherwise it would constitute a nuisance to other people in the area. You may find that this is quite restrictive. You will have to find alternative ways to dispose of manure, such as paying to have it taken away from time to time, or putting it in bags to put out on the side of the road for people to take away. In turn, this may restrict you to the type of bedding you can use. Most commercial manure distributors do not like shavings or alternative forms of bedding such as flax or paper. Therefore if you have a horse with a respiratory problem which has to be kept in a dust-free environment, you may find disposal of manure a problem and therefore find it difficult to cope with planning requirements.

Look at the provisions of the Environmental Protection Act 1990, Part 3 for guidance as to what would constitute a nuisance under that Act. The items listed there are what are termed 'statutory nuisances' – that is, situations set out in a law or 'statute' as being an unlawful nuisance. However, this does not mean that anything not set out in that list is *not* a nuisance. There can still be claims for 'private nuisances' – claims made under general law not using the Act, and if such a claim is made, the courts will look at whether the action claimed to be causing a nuisance is interfering with the 'enjoyment' of nearby land, or actually damaging it. This could cover having too many horses causing undue noise, or smell from a muckheap for instance.

If you do wish to apply for planning permission, you must apply to your local planning authority in whatever manner is set down by that particular authority. This is usually by means of a form provided by the authority. You will need to give full details of the proposed development, usually accompanied by a plan of the land and any other plans, drawings and information necessary to describe the development. You can apply for 'outline planning permission', which means you can get planning permission in principle to build something, but it may be subject to later and more detailed approvals.

You can also apply for renewal of planning permission which has previously been granted but building work has not yet begun, as long as it is within the time limit for the development to be built. Thus, you could buy a house with planning permission for stables which have not yet been built and could apply for renewal of that permission. It would be wise to ascertain with the local authority the prospect of such planning permission being renewed before you purchase the property, rather than assuming that the planning permission will automatically be renewed. Your conveyancing solicitor can do this for you.

You could also apply for variations of conditions of planning permission. You have to lodge the application with the local planning authority and there will be a fee unless the proposed development is 'permitted development'. Permitted development will be specified in the relevant Town and Country Planning General Development Order in force at the time. A register of applications is kept, containing copies of planning applications and eventual decisions. Planning permission applications

must be publicised, usually by displaying a copy of the planning application at a site on or near the land where the planning permission is
required and by advertising in the local paper. In some cases the owners
or occupiers of land or buildings adjoining the land of the proposed
development will be served with notice of the proposals as well.

Representations can be made to the planning authority by anyone who
wishes to comment on or object to the proposed development, or indeed
they could write in to support it. There is an appeal procedure if planning
permission is turned down.

Obviously this is only a brief outline of the procedure and there is much
more to planning permission than can be written here. Generally speaking the greater the development and the more impact it is likely to have on
the surrounding environment, the more it will be subject to scrutiny and
consultation before planning permission is granted.

If you find that you have become the owner of a structure that strictly
speaking needed planning permission but doesn't have it, or you have
built something that needed planning permission but you failed to get it,
it is possible in some cases to legalise the use by applying for Certificates
of Lawful Use or Lawful Development. Generally speaking, however,
unless you find yourself inadvertently in such a position, it is better to
obtain proper planning permission before the development takes place.

You may be tempted to build a stable or to start using, say, an agricultural barn to put your horses in without applying for any planning
permission. You may think that the planning authority will not notice.
This may work until you come to sell the house and it is discovered that
there is no planning permission for various buildings or the use of them;
or you may find that a neighbour is only too willing to bring your
development to the attention of the local planning authority, particularly
if you have fallen out. As ever, the advice has to be to keep everything on a
legal footing and ensure that you get proper permissions.

You would be obliged to keep your fencing in good order as horses that
are constantly escaping due to poor or inadequate fencing could not only
make you liable for any consequent damage caused by them, but could
also constitute a nuisance. Courts can order nuisances in whatever form to
be stopped or 'abated' by use of injunctions or other formal court orders.

The general rule is that it is your responsibility to fence in your horses,
not expect others to keep them out. If, due to your negligence, your horse
escapes and causes damage or injury, then you can be liable under the
Animals Act 1971 section 4, or if not under that Act then just generally in
negligence or nuisance. Section 4 says:

(1) Where livestock belonging to any other person strays onto land in
    ownership or occupation of another and –

(a) damage is done by the livestock to the land or to any property on it which is in the ownership or possession of the other person;

or

(b) any expenses are reasonably incurred by that other person in keeping the livestock while it cannot be restored to the person to whom it belongs or while it is detained in pursuance of section 7 of the Act or in ascertaining to whom it belongs;

the person to whom the livestock belongs is liable for the damage or expenses, except as otherwise provided by this Act.

(2) For the purposes of this section, any livestock belongs to the person in whose possession it is.'

This last clause means that the horse need not necessarily be your own; livery horses could be included if they could be said to be in your 'possession'.

Section 7 referred to in section 4 allows livestock to be detained where it has strayed onto other land. Such detention can only last for 48 hours unless the person detaining it reports it to the police – and it has to be to 'an officer in charge of a police station' – and to the person to whom the livestock belongs if they are known. To retrieve your horse, you have to pay in money – a cheque may not be acceptable – the amount of any claim for damages, or if there is no such claim, then the right to detain ceases when you arrive to claim your horse back.

If no-one claims the horse, the person detaining it can sell it in a market or at auction after 14 days, unless a claim for its return is still being sorted out – for example, if there is no agreement over the right amount to be paid, or if it is unclear who should be claiming the horse but there is someone who you think might be the owner, or if there is a claim under section 4. If the horse is sold, then the owner, if they come forward, will be entitled to the sale price, less costs of sale, the costs of any claim for damage or injury, and the cost of maintaining the horse while detained. Be careful if you hold onto a horse under this section; if you do not look after it properly and do not treat it with 'reasonable care' while it is in your possession, you could be liable for any damage or injury caused to it as a result.

No matter what the law appears to entitle you to do, be very careful before selling a horse under this provision. Alert the police and Horsewatch schemes, make detailed enquiries in the area with regard to lost horses, and keep the horse longer than 14 days if necessary until you are sure that you have done everything reasonable to track down the owner. Even after you have sold the horse, put the money into a separate bank account for a time until it is abundantly clear that no owner is going to come forward. However frustrated you might get if the same horses keep escaping onto your land, do not hold and sell them out of revenge.

As the owner of a horse, there are defences to section 4. You may not be liable if:

- The damage done is due wholly to the fault of the person suffering it – perhaps they let your horse out onto their land in the first place.
- The person suffering the damage voluntarily accepted the risk, for instance by allowing your horse to graze on their land.
- The horse was perfectly legally on a highway and strayed off onto the other land. It is difficult to put this in context; the usual example given is a herd of cows being taken from a field to the milking sheds using the road, where one of the cows strays into a garden and eats the plants. It could be that you are leading your horse along the road and he suddenly dives into a garden. As long as you were not negligent in allowing him to escape – perhaps he was suddenly frightened by a speeding motorbike – and you retrieve him as soon as possible from the garden, then you may have a defence to a claim.

You might, however, want to consider offering to pay for any damage nonetheless, even where you aren't entirely sure you should. This can be prudent from a neighbourly point of view and might also be cheaper than the legal fees involved in proving your 'innocence'.

It is no defence to say that the person who suffered the damage could have prevented the damage by putting up fencing, unless they do have a duty to put up such fencing and have failed to do so.

What happens if someone else lets your horses out or allows them to escape? You are unlikely to be liable if you have taken all reasonable precautions to secure your horses and, unbeknown to you, they are let out. In the case of *Jaundrill* v. *Gillett* (1996) (*Horse Law* (1996), Vol. 1, Iss. 1, *Horse and Hound* (1996) 11 Feb.), it was alleged that vandals had opened a gate and chased five horses onto a road, where they collided with a car, causing injury to the driver. The driver said that the owner of the horses was responsible because of the 'strict liability' (no need to prove fault – the fact that something has happened is enough for liability to be found) provisions of the Animals Act.

The driver succeeded with this argument at first, but the defendant owner appealed. The Court of Appeal granted the appeal. The judges said that the owner 'could not be responsible for the actions of people unknown to her, in this case described as vandals, who equally unknown to her let the horses out of what was a secure field'. There are no set guidelines as to what constitutes a 'secure field', but almost inevitably the word 'reasonable' will come into it somewhere. It probably does not mean a padlocked gate (this could be dangerous if emergency access was ever needed, say for veterinary attention) and security cameras, but if the fencing is weak or has gaps in it, then it may be held to not be secure. For instance, if your field has a right of way through it and you know people are going in and out constantly, it would be well worth investing in some sort of self-closing gate and solid fencing.

You should ensure that your fields are secure and are maintained to remain so, not only to ensure the safety of your own horses but also to enable you to defend a legal action.

You can keep horses on unfenced land provided it is 'common land' in the legal sense of the term and you have the right to put your horses there. If they then stray off that land, you may not be liable for any damage caused – section 8(2) of the Animals Act. The reasoning is that common land cannot be fenced by law, so it is unfair to hold people liable if horses stray from an area where they are not allowed to be fenced in anyway. It is not negligent to allow horses to graze on unfenced land in this way, but it is definitely not recommended. However legal it may be, it is not safe. If you have to keep horses in this way, then try tethering.

Tethering

It is not illegal to tether, but you could find yourself liable under the Cruel Tethering Act 1988 if the tethering causes unnecessary suffering. The British Horse Society produce a leaflet with guidelines for tethering which in outline are:

- Provide adequate clean water, grazing or forage, shelter, shade and exercise.
- Do not tether in extreme weather – rain, cold, heatwaves, etc. – unless you can provide shelter and/or shade.
- Remove manure regularly.
- Consider the suitability of your horse for tethering. Is it old, highly strung, young or a mare in season? If so, it should not really be tethered.
- Do not allow your horse to be tethered unsupervised.
- Inspect the horse at least once a day and preferably more.
- Use a suitable site – no hazards, rubbish or uneven ground.
- Use a comfortable soft wide leather strap or headcollar with a swivel chain of suitable weight and length, not too heavy such that it drags on the horse. Check the horse regularly for sores or rubbing. In the case of *RSPCA* v. *Allen* (1996), Mr Allen was fined £400 and banned from keeping a horse for five years after being convicted of an offence under

the Cruel Tethering Act. A mare he owned was found to have a 2 in deep wound behind her ears where the tether had been too tight and had rubbed.

• Make sure your horse is suitably vaccinated and wormed regularly.

Tethering should be a last resort and if the horse has to be kept like this permanently or long term, you should consider whether you should be keeping the horse. Tethering may be suitable for, say, overnight stays on holiday or if the horse belongs to a group constantly on the move as a way of life, where there is constant supervision and change of grazing, but it is not really an acceptable way of keeping a horse today. It may be that your horse has to be tethered for health reasons – you may need to restrict his grazing, for instance. This can be acceptable as long as good management practices are adhered to; it is horses kept tethered for long periods in unsuitable conditions that are the concern.

Under section 155 of the Highways Act 1980, it is an offence for a horse to be found straying on or lying in or at the side of a highway, unless the highway is going across common, waste or unenclosed land.

Control of ragwort

One point you might like to take note as a horse owner is the control of ragwort in your fields. Under the Weeds Act 1959, ragwort is an 'injurious weed' and one that on agricultural land must be controlled. This may not apply to you as a horse owner in terms of strict law, as you may not be on agricultural land, but clearly it would be good husbandry to comply with its eradication. If you find that you are clearing your grazing of it, but you are constantly suffering re-infestation from sources where the ragwort should be cleared, then you could try approaching the owner of the land to try to get them to put in place an eradication and control programme. Unfortunately there is no obvious other way – only perhaps an action for nuisance, which would be costly and difficult to prove.

If the ragwort is on the roads, then you should advise your local authority or the Highways Agency through the County Council Highways Engineers Maintenance Department whose number will be in your local telephone directory. Of course, not only ragwort is covered by the Weeds Act 1959, but it is the plant that is most likely to appear and cause injury to your horses. It is highly toxic and is even more dangerous dried than fresh. It can be controlled by spraying in April to early June but this does mean that you will not be able to use the ground for grazing until all the sprayed plants have died and been cleared out. You may also find that if you blanket spray you will kill other plants that do no harm to your horse and may in fact be beneficial. Another option is to dig ragwort out plant by plant, removing the entire plant including the roots. This can be done on a plant by plant basis if there is only a small amount, or by mechanical means if there are a large number. Cutting the plants back or mowing them may just encourage them to grow even more vigorously. Once dug out the plants should be comprehensively burnt and the remains not used for fertiliser-type purposes. A lot of people graze sheep with horses but do remember that ragwort is toxic to sheep as well.

It may also be a good practical measure to put up fencing to keep your horse away from poisonous plants and trees. In an ideal world, you would not put horses near yew trees or poisonous hedges, but sometimes there is no choice. Sometimes it is the landowner's responsibility to remove toxic plants or ensure they are not in the horses' reach, and if you have a formal arrangement than you could make provision in that for the landowner to be responsible. However, many of us have much more haphazard or loose arrangements. Would you rather spend money on fencing and still have a horse, or do you want to spend your time and money arguing over who should have done what after you've buried the horse?

Do, however make sure if you put up fencing yourself that it does the job adequately. Although fencing your horse out is a practical move, you could be depriving yourself of any rights you may have, in the event of anything untoward happening, against someone else who should have taken responsibility, the argument being that you have effectively taken responsibility yourself.

Liability to rates

You will have to pay rates on certain buildings whether you are a riding stable, a livery stable or have horses at home. There are exemptions for agricultural animals but, as mentioned earlier, horses are not classed as agricultural livestock in this context. The 'occupier' of the land is liable for the rates. The occupier may not be the owner of the land, they may be the tenant. In the case of a riding school licence under the Riding Establishments Acts, the occupier may not necessarily be the licence holder. Rates are payable on the 'rateable value' of the building and this is a matter of evidence of value, which can be very subjective. If you do not inform the local authority of a change of use or a development, and the building or development becomes rateable, then they may not notice for a while but rates can be backdated to when they should have been paid. There appears to be no duty to inform the local authority of a change of use or a development but it is best to play safe and inform them. If you fail to inform the local authority due to a genuine oversight or lack of realisation that you should be paying rates, but you do inform them as soon as possible when you find out, then the local authority may be more sympathetic than if they suspect you have deliberately concealed the fact that you should pay rates in order to avoid payment.

Stables and buildings are not agricultural buildings and are liable to rates, but land used solely or predominantly for grazing horses may well be exempt agricultural land and not liable for rates. You may think that you can escape paying rates by saying that the buildings that house your horses are in fact agricultural buildings and therefore not liable to rates. This is not so. You have to look at what the buildings are currently used for. Your stables may well be former pig units, but if they have horses in them now they are stables and will be liable for rates.

You will be liable for rates whether you operate commercially or privately. The liability to pay rates does not depend on whether or not you make a profit from the use of the buildings. Also, do not think because you do not need planning permission for a building that it is automatically not liable to rates. It may not be, if you build a stable in what counts for legal purposes as your garden and the stables are for your personal and private use and not for business use; those stables may then be included in the overall rateable value of the house and garden in the same way that a garage might be looked on as part of the house. Therefore the stables would not be rated separately, although they would be taken into account.

Your house will have a Council Tax banding and the amount you pay will depend on which band you are in. The bands are governed by the value of the house. The Council Tax band you are in stays the same until the house is sold, no matter how much the house is improved or added to during your occupancy. Therefore, when buying a property you may find that it is Band A for Council Tax purposes, meaning that you think you will not have to pay very much, but the property might have been improved during the occupancy of the owners and when you move in might jump up to a different band, which will be much more expensive.

There is a special rateable relief available for studs whereby the rateable value can be reduced by an amount specified by the Secretary of State from time to time. To qualify, the buildings housing the animals must be used for the breeding and/or rearing of horses and ponies and must be occupied, together with any agricultural land or agricultural building. The land must be more than 2 hectares in extent.

Chapter 9
Saddlers and Saddle Fitters

Once you've bought your horse and installed him in his new home, you'll want to ride. That means you'll need tack.

When considering buying a new saddle, do remember that saddlers, master or otherwise, are not necessarily saddle fitters, although they can be. Most complaints arise from the fitting of the saddle rather than from the saddle itself. You may purchase a saddle which is perfectly made in all respects, but it will be of no use if it doesn't fit your horse. This will not usually be the saddler's fault, unless she or he has advised on fitting the saddle or has measured up for the saddle and either measured incorrectly or made the saddle incorrectly.

The same principles apply to bridles and rugs or any equipment either made to measure or fitted by someone who is qualified to do so, or who holds themselves out as being qualified to do so. It doesn't matter if someone doesn't have any recognised training or qualifications (this applies in any area, not just saddle fitting). If they say they are capable of properly making or fitting equipment (and saddles are probably the biggest area for this), they are 'holding themselves out' as having that particular skill, and they will be expected to reach the same standard as someone who does have recognised qualifications in that skill. They cannot expect to work to a lower standard or make more mistakes and then escape by pleading that they are not qualified to make or fit saddles – they've just been doing it for a long time or picked it up from someone else, but they haven't passed any exams. This is not to say that everyone who has qualifications will be excellent, whereas someone with experience but no formal qualifications should not be used. It is just that qualifications at least give some indication of the level of expertise that the person has, and show that the person has been committed enough to bother going through qualification procedures.

Saddles bought where one party is a business and the other is a private individual are governed by the Sale of Goods Act 1979 as amended by the Sale and Supply of Goods Act 1984. Briefly, there is an implied term that the goods are satisfactory and will be fit for their purpose. An implied term is a term of a contract that is implied to be there by law, whether or not a contract has it included. The Act also applies to second-hand saddles and other used items which, even though they have been used, can still be defective in other ways. For instance, a broken tree is a defect whether it is in a new saddle or a third-hand saddle. However, if a particular defect is brought to your attention before sale and you buy the saddle with full knowledge of that defect, you can't then rely on that defect to take it back as defective.

If you need a particular sort of item or it is going to be used for a specific purpose, and you make your requirements and/or the purpose known to the seller, then if it is reasonable for you to do so you can rely on their assurance that it is that item and/or it is fit for the purpose expressed. If it later proves not to be so, you can take it back. When would it be reasonable for you to rely on someone else's assurance? Usually this would be if you have no specialist knowledge yourself, or no knowledge specialist or otherwise of the product you are considering buying, but each case will depend on its own facts and on who said what to whom.

If you are buying a saddle as a private individual from another private individual, then the Act does not apply and you should examine the saddle carefully for any defects. Once you have bought the item it is unlikely that you would be able to return it even if defective, particularly if you had had the opportunity to inspect it; and it would be uneconomic to litigate in most cases. You should not buy a saddle sight unseen and it is not recommended either that you make a major purchase like a saddle at an auction, although rugs, bits, bridles, headcollars, etc. are usually all right as they are more easily fitted and tend to be more flexible on the number of horses they will fit. There is also considerably less chance of them causing a problem if they do not fit exactly.

Incorrect or defective saddles

If the saddle or other equipment you have bought (the example of a saddle will be used as that is the most common) is incorrect or defective when received, then it should be possible to return it if bought commercially and get your money back. If it is incorrect, e.g. a 17 in saddle has been made rather than the 18 in ordered, even if there is nothing wrong with it as a saddle, it will still not be the saddle you contracted for. You can therefore return it as it is not as per contract. If you ordered a black saddle and a brown one arrives, the same applies.

A useful tip is to buy items with a credit card (*not* a debit card) if you have one. If you do this and the item you have bought is faulty, or the company or shop you bought it from goes bankrupt before it delivers the goods, you can claim your money back from the credit card company rather than the shop or company if they are being difficult. This is because under the Consumer Credit Act 1974, both the credit card company and the shop or company are liable for transactions made by credit card. It only applies to goods worth over £100 and up to £30,000, but will still apply if you are only leaving a deposit on an item worth that much.

You must return the item within a reasonable time – and this will differ according to the circumstances. Some defects might take a little time to show up. In these circumstances, you should take the item back as soon as you are aware of the defect or even if you just suspect there is one. If the defect is obvious, e.g. the saddle is the wrong colour, then there is nothing to stop you returning the item immediately. You can see what is wrong straightaway and there is no good reason for you to keep it for any length of time. You cannot expect to use a saddle for some months and then take it back saying it is the wrong colour. You will almost certainly be deemed to have accepted the saddle as it is and to have lost your right to return it and get your money back or even exchange it.

Difficulties arise where the saddle is not quite as you ordered but is not completely wrong. Say, for instance, you ordered a brown saddle and you get a brown saddle, but it is two shades darker than the leather you saw when you ordered it. Can you return it or refuse to take it? It can depend on whether there is a 'fundamental breach of contract'. Was it absolutely essential that the saddle was a particular shade of brown and did you make this clear on ordering? You may for instance have all your other equipment in a particular colour and therefore it was vital that your new saddle matched. This may be especially important with sponsor's colours. If, on the other hand, the exact colour is unimportant except that you thought it was going to be a little lighter than it was, then the breach may not be so severe as to be 'fundamental' to the whole contract. You may not be able to take it back as of right, assuming there is nothing else wrong with it, but you might perhaps get it a little cheaper if you point out the discrepancy. Something of that nature would rarely if ever be worth taking to formal litigation.

If the item is defective rather than incorrect and the defect goes on to cause an injury to you or the horse, then there may be a claim under the Consumer Protection Act 1987, as well as a claim under the normal contract principles of the item being as per contract, of satisfactory quality and reasonably fit for its purpose. The good point about the Consumer Protection Act is that if you can prove there is a defect and it has caused injury, then there is in legal terms almost a 'strict liability'.

Strict liability is where someone is found to be at fault for doing something, even where they didn't mean to or didn't realise they had done something legally wrong. Usually, with strict liability offences there is no defence whatsoever; the fact that the wrong has been done is enough. Under the Consumer Protection Act, however, there is a tiny get-out clause: if the manufacturer of the item could not possibly have known of the defect, then they may escape liability. But it is not enough not to have known of the defect, it must actually have been impossible to know about it, usually because the knowledge was not there. If it was there, then the manufacturers will usually be expected to know about it, however obscure. The manufacturers will also not be able to claim that the item was not dangerous or that they didn't know it was dangerous because there had been no previous accidents caused by this defect. There doesn't have to be. The fact that the defect exists is enough (*Abouzaid* v. *Mothercare* 2001, *The Times*, 20 February).

As an example, if a saddle was made with a defective type of stirrup leather holder, and the defect meant that the leather was always going to slip off, then the whole saddle might be seen as defective as it would not be safe to use a saddle where the leathers slip off. You could return it as being not of satisfactory quality and not fit for its purpose under the Sale of Goods Act. If the leather did come off and as result you were injured, you could possibly make a claim under the Consumer Protection Act. You could do both as alternatives. Do remember that under the Consumer Protection Act there would have to be an injury. If the leather came off, but nothing happened, then there would be nothing to claim for, although you could still take the saddle back and try and get your money back or an exchange if the leathers kept slipping off.

Fitting the saddle

Of course, the seller will not be able to guarantee that the saddle, whether bought commercially or privately, will fit your horse. This is where you will need the services of the saddle fitter, who may be the person who sold you the saddle, or someone completely different.

There is a professional saddle-fitting qualification set up by the Society of Master Saddlers. There is a strict code of conduct and agreed fitting procedure, and qualified saddle fitters must have a knowledge of the horse's anatomy and the purpose that the horse is used for, and be able to assess the rider's build, needs, standards of riding and experience. For instance, very experienced showjumpers may well be able to cope with a close contact saddle, but it would not suit an inexperienced rider. Under the code of conduct, a saddle fitter must keep records of the saddle fitting.

Qualified saddle fitters must re-register annually and undertake a saddle-fitting refresher course every two years. A saddle-fitter will not necessarily make saddles but will be concerned as to whether or not the saddle you have, whether you have already bought it or are buying it from the fitter, does fit. The saddle fitter may bring a selection of saddles for you to choose from. There is again a contract where the implied terms of reasonable skill and care apply. The usual principles apply. If a saddle fitter fails in his duty and as a result injury or financial loss occurs, you may have a legitimate complaint. Once again, if the matter becomes hotly contested, i.e. there are allegations that not only has the saddle been incorrectly fitted but it has also caused substantial damage to your horse, then you will probably need to consult a solicitor. Expert evidence would almost certainly be needed to prove your case as claimant, and possibly even to defend it; a saddler/fitter might be able to give evidence in a quasi-expert role on their own behalf.

However, before you get to that stage, if you contact the Society of Master Saddlers they may be willing to act as mediator between the saddler/fitter and yourself and try and resolve the dispute that way. You could both agree to abide by the Society's decision.

As ever, it is to be hoped that complaints and potential claims, particularly those of a relatively small financial value, can be sorted out amicably before costs and tempers escalate.

Chapter 10
Riding Horses on the Road

Horses are traffic just as much as cars, and the Highway Code specifically refers to recommendations for horses on the road and for driver reactions. It should be remembered that the Highway Code is only a guide and is not law in the strict sense of the word, although of course it is a very persuasive guide. Drivers have a duty to a horse and rider but equally riders have a duty to themselves and others on the road. Drivers cannot expect a horse to behave perfectly all the time, as seen in the case of *Carryfast Ltd* v. *Hack* (1981) (RTR 464) where a driver was held negligent for failing to slow down and give a wide berth to a horse 'messing about' on the road. On the other hand, as a rider you cannot expect to take out a horse that you cannot control or that is dangerous in traffic, and expect drivers to know this and make the necessary allowances.

Paragraphs 139, 190 and 191 of the Highway Code give motorists some general guidance on driving in the vicinity of animals, horses and riders, such as slowing down and not sounding the horn. Riders should look at paragraphs 35–41, which suggest general tips for safe riding.

You must do your best to be as safe, visible (paragraphs 35 and 36 of the Highway Code) and as in control of your horse as possible. If you are a driver you should expect the unexpected, especially on country roads. You should slow down, particularly around corners and when you are approaching horses. Pass wide and slowly around horses. Flashing your lights, revving your engine, squeezing past close to a horse and driving practically on a horse's heels will not help the situation or make the rider go any faster if it is not safe to do so. The Highway Code particularly warns against this (paragraphs 190 and 191). As a driver, have you ever seen the damage a horse can do if it sits on a car? If a horse lands on the roof it can very easily depress the roof to the floor, crushing you if you happen to be in the way.

Riders should not, however, dawdle along chatting, two abreast, allowing a frustrated line of cars to build up behind. When out riding keep a careful watch on the traffic situation and get into single file and move your horse into a space or a gateway, if possible, to let built-up traffic pass. Do remember that you are not allowed to ride horses on the pavement, on footpaths or in the cycle lane (Highways Act 1835, section 72).

There are all sorts of myths about riders and horses being 'allowed' to take up the road to the extent of the width of one car. This is not so. You can ride two abreast; it is not illegal to do so but it can be unsafe, e.g. on corners. This does in some cases create a contradiction as you are told to ride a young horse with an older, safe horse between it and the traffic, and of course when you are leading a horse the person should be between the horse and the traffic. Use common sense. If you need to ride two abreast try to stick to wide roads where you will be visible for a long way ahead. The Highway Code specifically warns drivers to be aware of riders and of riders leading two abreast (paragraph 191). Is there a horse and rider warning triangle roadsign where you ride? If not, consider asking the local highway authority to put one up in an area where there are a number of horses and riders or there is a riding school. It may not stop all accidents, but at least if there is an accident a driver might find it difficult to say he or she did not realise there might be horses on the road.

If leading a horse use a bridle, pass the reins through the bit to the right side and lead the horse on your left, on the left-hand side of the road. Check whether your insurance policy covers you when you are leading and if so, whether there is a maximum number of horses you can lead – usually only one.

Child riders

Children under 14 must wear a riding helmet which complies with the appropriate safety standards in force at the time for hats and helmets and the Horses (Protective Headgear for Young Riders) Regulations 1992. Older riders are recommended to do the same. In both cases the helmet should be fastened securely. Wearing of body protectors is not so regulated although the standards of body protectors are; you may wish to wear one for added protection.

It must be for parents to decide when their children should go out on their own on horses or ponies, or alternatively it is the responsiblity of others who are in charge of the riding arrangements at the time, for instance riding school instructors or trek leaders. They should make an assessment of when it is safe to let a child out on their own and should ensure that the horse is as safe as possible. You might ask what would happen if you did your assessment and thought all was well, but the child still had an accident. It is likely that those making the assessment would not be liable if their assessment had been made reasonably. If the assessment was clearly wrong, then it might be a different matter.

For instance, if you are aware that the child is very capable and is riding a horse they have been riding for a long time and which has never misbehaved in traffic, and the roads are quiet, then it is reasonable to assume that all will be well barring unforeseen circumstances. If on the other hand you assess a child who has only been riding three or four times, on a horse they have never ridden before, as safe to go out on a road, then your assessment is clearly unreasonable. The fact that you have made an assessment will not protect you; the outcome of the assessment has to be reasonable.

Safety clothing and equipment

Livery yard owners are unlikely to be responsible for riders going out from their yard, unless of course for some reason the livery yard owner has supplied the horse, but it may damage your reputation as a yard owner if horses from your yard attract a continual stream of complaints or are the cause of accidents. It is possible that you could become liable if you continue to let dangerous or careless riders carry on. You could make it a condition of your livery contract that hats and other safety equipment are to be worn or used at all times when in the yard, whether with the livery's own horse or not. What your adult liveries choose to do off the yard is largely up to them.

You should always wear reflective gear such as a bib or reflective jacket and your horse should wear some reflective clothing as well. There is an enormous amount of reflective equipment available on the market, including rain sheets, nose and brow band covers, exercise sheets, fetlock bands and tail bandages.

Always remember to check your tack for safety before you set out. Do not leave repairs undone. If in doubt then don't ride until you have had your tack repaired or replaced.

Riding at night

Do not ride out at dusk or at night if you can avoid it. It is not illegal but can be dangerous. If you have to ride or lead at night – say your horse has gone lame and you are later home than you thought, then walk on the outside of your horse. As a precaution, try and carry some sort of reflective gear with you if you are not already wearing it, so that you can put it on when needed. Invest in stirrup lights or a light to carry; white light goes to the front, red to the rear. If there is more than one of you, try and place a light coloured horse at the rear or on the outside if you have to ride or lead two abreast.

Riding in groups

You should never ride more than two abreast in anything other than open countryside and try not to ride in a larger group than eight if it can be avoided. These are British Horse Society recommendations. They are not saying that it is always acceptable to ride in a group of eight horses; they are saying that a maximum of eight should be aimed for. If in some circumstances it is prudent to ride in a group of less than eight, that is what should be done. It might be acceptable to ride in a larger group depending on countryside, horse temperaments and riding ability – for example, a hunt does not restrict itself to eight members of the field.

If you are riding in a group, you should ride in single file, or in pairs if it is safe to do so. There should be a responsible ride leader over 16 years of age at the front and preferably a ride 'bringer-up' at the back. The group should keep close together and make sure every member understands signals, both formal road signals and pre-arranged signals or instructions organised by the ride leaders in case of a problem.

Traffic regulations

Horses and riders are subject to traffic regulations. Horses and riders are allowed on any road (even surprisingly a dual carriageway) except motorways. You must observe traffic regulations such as traffic lights, give way signs, zebra crossings, etc. in the same way as cars. On roundabouts, drivers should be especially on the lookout for horses and riders as they can stay in the left-hand lane while signalling right if they are going right round a roundabout. A car would most likely be in the right-hand lane for the same purpose.

As a rider, you must be very careful to give clear signals in good time and to show courtesy at all times to other road users. The Highway Code suggests that you keep both hands on the reins at all times. However, the British Horse Society suggests you raise a hand to thank drivers. Is this then negligent? It might be if you are on a difficult horse where control takes priority over courtesy; try a nod of thanks instead, or have a tabard made with 'Thank you for slowing down' printed on it. Drivers should be aware that it is not always possible for a rider to acknowledge them; a nervous rider may feel unsafe taking a hand off the reins, but that doesn't mean that riders are not grateful for drivers' consideration.

Insurance

It is not compulsory to have insurance to ride on the roads, although there is some debate as to whether it should be. If a car driver is the cause of an accident and injures you, the rider, then they will nearly always have insurance against which you can claim for your injuries and financial losses. However, if you are the cause of the accident and the car driver is completely blameless, then they may be advised against pursuing a claim against you if you are not insured, particularly if there are no other assets. If you do have assets – such as a house which belongs to you (even if it is mortgaged), a sum of money in the bank or building society, cars, land, equipment or even sometimes horses – then any judgment for compensation can in some circumstances be enforced against these assets. This would mean that the assets would be sold and the money used to pay compensation. In the case of a house, something called a 'charge' would be put against it. This means that the house may not be required to be sold immediately to pay compensation, but when it is sold, part or perhaps all of the proceeds will go towards paying the compensation. In extreme cases, sale of the assets including the house can be enforced. It is strongly recommended that you are insured. It is another expense each year but perhaps you really don't need five different supplements for your horse or yet another pair of jodhpurs for yourself.

Road safety test

You do not have to pass any test to be allowed on the roads with a horse, but again it is strongly recommended that you take the British Horse Society Riders and Road Safety Test. This will not only teach you safe riding on the roads, but if you are involved in an accident it could be good evidence on your part that you were and are a conscientious rider, taking all precautions to be safe on the road and avoid an accident. This would be as long as you were riding in accordance with the recommendations of the test, of course. There are also financial advantages to taking the test. Many insurers will offer reduced premiums or increased cover for those successfully passing the test who are then involved in an accident while adhering to the test recommendations. The British Horse Society produces booklets on riding and road safety and a booklet giving a list of test dates for the year. It is well worth getting these and putting yourself through the test with updates from time to time. But do remember that it will be you who has taken the test, not your horse. Being able to pass a test in controlled conditions does not mean you can relax and assume your horse is now totally safe on roads, no matter what.

Weather conditions

Watch the weather. Horses can slip in icy conditions, and fog will make it difficult to see you. Consider whether you should go out at all. You might, at least, be contributorily negligent if you go out in dangerous conditions and then are involved in an accident, for instance because of the horse slipping on ice and falling in front of a car. Sunny weather is no guarantee of safety. Drivers can be blinded by the sun on rounding a corner and you can be tempted on sunny days not to wear reflective gear. Sometimes this means that you will blend into the background.

Horse-drawn vehicles

All these comments apply equally to horse-drawn vehicles. Check the driving harness, ensure your horse is safe and well-trained especially in traffic, ensure that you can be seen, and be courteous – traffic can less easily pass a horse and trap than a single horse. There is an interesting case relating to horse-drawn vehicles, which has its amusing side but is not to be relied upon as a defence! The case is *R* v. *Beard and Bowman* (1995) (*Horse Law* (1996) Vol. 1, Iss. 1). The *R* indicates it is a criminal prosecution with the *R* standing for Regina, i.e. the Crown. It is the Crown, through the Crown Prosecution Service, which prosecutes, not, as some people think, the police, although they can make recommendations.

In this particular case, the two defendants were apparently trotting along with separate horses and trotting carts, seemingly at an innocent jog trot. A police car pulled alongside with the police driver giving hand signals to the effect that they should stop. The drivers were apparently slowing their horses up when the police car put on its blue light and began to pull in front of the horses and carts. Startled, the horses began to trot faster. The police driver then switched on the car's siren! The poor horses were quite overcome by this and bolted, only to the surprise perhaps of the police officer. The defendants were charged with the wonderfully ancient-sounding offence of 'furiously driving a carriage', but were, quite sensibly it seems, acquitted.

Don't drink and ride

Finally, do remember that it is an offence to be drunk in charge of a horse. There are numerous old boys' tales of horses plodding quietly home from the local ale house with their masters falling asleep on their backs or in the driving seat, having consumed rather too many pints of the local alcoholic speciality. Section 12 of the Licensing Act 1872 states that it is an offence to be in charge of any carriage, horse or indeed cattle on any highway or public place when drunk. For the purpose of this offence, a breathalyser is not used to decide whether someone is 'drunk'; it can be much less scientific and depend more on observation of whether you appear to be affected by alcohol. The case of *R* v. *Matthew Clark* (1997) (*Horse Law* Vol. 2, Iss. 2, *The Times*, 30 Jan.) suggests that under the case of *Lanhan* v. *Richmond* (1984) (148 JP 737), you would be regarded as 'drunk' if you had 'lost the power of self control' due to being drunk. It is not quite clear how this would be interpreted, but it is strongly suggested that you don't drink and ride any more than you should drink and drive.

Chapter 11
Bridleways and Tracks

You will not want to ride your horse only on the road; indeed you will probably want to keep off the road as much as possible, using it only as a means of access to bridleways or other permitted rides. The provision of off-road hacking varies greatly from county to county. The strength of local pressure groups can greatly affect the provision of off-road riding, private courses, horse crossings in new developments, etc. The British Horse Society are very keen to promote bridleways and have a network of access officers across the country who in turn liaise with designated rights of way and access representatives in local riding clubs. If you have a query with regard to a bridleway – does it exist, can it be diverted, can a footpath be upgraded, etc. – a very good place to start would be the British Horse Society who can give you the name and contact details of your local area access officer.

The law is complicated and involves the interaction of several different Acts, but the common law (law that is not written down in specific Acts) is also used. One of the problems with countryside access is that a number of groups are all competing for the right to use scarce resources and there can be a conflict between their requirements. Ramblers do not necessarily want to find themselves with a horse cantering towards them, nor do they want to walk on a muddy path churned up by hooves, while riders may find it difficult to canter anywhere if paths are full of people ambling along. Neither ramblers nor riders want motorbikes or off-road vehicles to use the same tracks as they do, because of the damage caused, but those groups will say they have as much right as riders or ramblers to use certain paths. Cyclists will want a firm surface to ride on, but horse riders may not want this as it will be too hard on their horses' legs. Landowners may not want anyone on their land at all, although it does seem that farmers and landowners are slowly realising the commercial prospects of opening up their land and are developing rides to be used on payment of a regular fee, so perhaps this will be a partial solution. That should not mean that we give up campaigning for bridleways to be identified, opened and maintained. Riders would not want to reach a position where they are the only group forced to pay for something which others enjoy as a right. Nevertheless, 'toll rides' as they are becoming known, do offer a safe and enjoyable riding facility and can be well worth the fee per year. Even access to a small area can mean that reaching a much wider area is made possible.

South Eastern Toll Rides (01233 850320) were the first to set up this idea and can provide an information pack on setting up these rides – do offer to pay, or at least send an S.A.E! Grants are sometimes available for these schemes. Landowners should be aware that business rates are payable on the ride, but it can be possible to set up a charity to provide some rate relief, and negotiation with the local council can sometimes be possible, especially where the community amenity benefit can be stressed. Part of the fee payable by the riders will usually go to the landowner, with part withheld for maintenance. A proper agreement should be drawn up between riders and landowners, and licences granted. You will need a way of identifying licence holders – a coloured armband perhaps – and the ride will need policing, but not in too authoritarian a manner. It will take some organisation and commitment to set up and run toll rides and both sides have to show goodwill, but it has to be worth it – income for landowners and safe hacks for riders. SETR are even considering whether it would be possible to have some sort of countrywide network or franchise operation to expand the scheme.

Also, watch out for provisions of the 'right to roam' law (Countryside and Rights of Way Act 2000). Much of it is not yet in force and it is not clear how the proposed rights of access to the countryside will work practically.

Rights of way

Rights of way generally fall into three categories:

- Byways open to all traffic (BOATS). A byway open to all traffic means a highway over which the public has a right of way for vehicular and all other kinds of traffic, but which is mainly used by the public as a footpath and bridleway.
- Footpaths – which are unclassified county roads, field roads and green lanes (UCRS). A footpath means a highway over which the public has a right of way on foot only, but it does not include a highway at the side of a public road.
- Bridleways – (defined in s329 Highways Act 1980) which means highways over which the public has the following, but no other rights of way:
  - a right of way on foot and a right of way on horseback; or

–   leading a horse with or without the right to drive animals of any description along the highway.

If you see the description 'public path', this can mean a highway which is either a footpath or a bridleway. These are roads used as a public path (shortened to 'RUPPs') and you will often see this definition on older maps; it is no longer permitted and the path has to be more specifically defined. The above definitions will be found in the Wildlife and Countryside Act 1981 section 54. The British Horse Society recommend the Ordnance Survey 1:250000 maps, the Pathfinder Series, for identifying bridleways, which will generally be shown as a line of green dashes.

Definitive map

If you want to find out more about bridleways in your area, you need to go to the 'definitive map' which is held by the highway authority, with copies usually also available in County Council offices, local authority offices and possibly libraries. The map can be inspected by the public at no charge, although it is usually best to ring up and make an appointment to view to make sure that there is someone available to let you have access to the map. The background to this map, which purports to be the final and definitive map showing all rights of way, is that under the National Parks and Access to the Countryside Act 1949, County Councils were required to map out their areas and show public rights of way. This was a lengthy process, but eventually the map was completed. The Wildlife and Countryside Act 1981 repealed this Act and under the new Act, the map must be kept up to date (section 53 of the Act) and continually reviewed and altered to reflect changes in rights of way.

Where there is a definitive map in existence, it is conclusive evidence that at the 'relevant date' (what this is can differ) the footpaths, bridleways, byways open to all traffic, public paths and highways shown were in existence to a certain extent (Wildlife and Countryside Act 1981, section 56(1). For instance, with reference to bridleways, the map is evidence that there was 'a highway over which the public had a right of way on foot and the right of way on horseback or leading a horse, but without prejudice as to whether the public had any other right of way'. This means that there may be further rights, e.g. the right to drive a vehicle down such a bridleway, but the map will not tell you that. Footpaths are evidence that the public has a right of way on foot, but no other right of way. Very often, horse riders wish to challenge this and will want to prove that the road identified and classified as a footpath is in fact a bridleway and therefore could be used by horse riders; or you may wish to have a right of way identified as a bridleway if there is evidence to show that it should be.

The Highways Act 1986 section 31 says that where 'a way over land... has been actually enjoyed by the public *as of right* and without interruption for a period of 20 years, the way is deemed to have been dedicated as a highway unless there is sufficient evidence there was no intention during that period to dedicate.' With bridleways, horses and riders must have used the path. Evidence of use by walkers is not evidence of a bridleway although evidence of use by cyclists could be. This is because cyclists are allowed to use bridleways but evidence of use by cyclists alone is not enough.

The 20 year period is counted backwards from when the question of whether or not the public have a right to use that path is raised. There is no specific way in which the question has to be raised – riders might suddenly find a locked gate has been put in place, or they have been asked to leave a path they have been using for years. The intention not to dedicate land for use as a path can be fulfilled by the erection of a visible notice to that effect. If a notice like this appears, it would constitute the question being raised. If the path is officially closed for at least one day a year, this can indicate a clear intention not to dedicate a path. Note that this only applies to land where the public have a *right* in the first place to go over it. Being given permission to ride over land is not the same as having the right to do so.

Seeking changes to the map

To challenge the definitive map and have it changed or added to can be a very long and intensive business, requiring careful gathering of evidence and an application to the 'surveying authority' – the County Council, Metropolitan and District Council or London Borough Council whose jurisdiction includes the area where the path is situated. The application will be in a particular form as set down by regulations made by the Secretary of State. Ask at your local council office for details. Evidence can be anything relevant in support, for instance, old maps, drawings, plans, statements, sworn witness statements (in the form of a statutory declaration) from people who remember using the rights of way on horseback – a sample questionnaire drawn up by the Ramblers' Association is produced by the British Horse Society and available on request from them – letters, minutes of Parish Council meetings, archive material, even an old painting showing the use of a path.

If you are seeking to challenge the classification or existence of a bridleway, it is recommended that you enlist the help of the British Horse Society or the Country Land and Business Association. It is also recommended that a liaison group is formed to try and share the work, as much work is involved and it is not fair to expect one person to take on the whole burden, particularly where a success would benefit many people. Remember that you are not looking to upgrade footpaths to bridleways, except by consent of the landowner or the local authority; you are trying to show that the path was incorrectly classified or missed off the map in the first place and is in fact a bridleway and should have been shown as such.

Once you have completed the lengthy task of compiling your evidence, you will need to make your application and serve notice of it to every owner and occupier, e.g. a tenant of the land to which your application relates. If you don't know who these people are, you can ask the council for permission to notify them by leaving a notice on the path in question. The British Horse Society suggests that you take photographs of the notices placed in position, using a camera which shows the date on the photographs to show when they were taken, and have the photographs signed by a witness.

You must also serve a 'Certificate of Compliance' on the relevant authority, e.g. the County Council. You can get this form from them.

The authority then have to investigate your application, consult with the local authority – usually a Parish Council – and make a decision as to whether to grant your application and order that the definitive map be altered to show the status of the path as a bridleway. They must tell you their decision. There is a right of appeal to the Secretary of State for the Department of the Environment, Food and Rural Affairs (DEFRA).

Before making the order, the relevant council must publicise the decision to make the 'Modification Order' – literally the order modifying the status of the path – describing the general effects of the order and the fact that it has been made, subject to confirmation. The council must give details of a place in the area of the land to which the order relates where a copy of the order can be inspected and copied, and must give a time, usually not less than 42 days from the date of the publication of the order, for representations and objections to be made. (Don't forget that applications can be made saying that bridleways are in fact footpaths, so if as a rider you see such a notice you may want to make representations and object.) The relevant authority must publish a notice to the same effect in a newspaper local to the area where the land is, and must serve notice on various people – the owners and occupiers of the land, the local authority for that land, anyone who has paid to be notified of such orders and anyone else who has a right to know or who the authority think should be notified. The notice should also be placed at the ends of the path affected, at the council offices and 'such other place as the Authority thinks appropriate'. These are therefore the places you need to look to see if there are any changes planned. Your local riding club might want to pay to be kept informed as at least you would then know of any proposed changes.

This all sounds straightforward but can be very complicated. If objections are received, there may have to be a local public enquiry. The council has 12 months in which to make a decision, so it can be a long business. You should ensure that the council is kept focused on the investigation by making regular enquiries as to progress. If a decision has not been made within 12 months, you should write to the Secretary of State for the Department of the Environment, Food and Rural Affairs (DEFRA) or its current equivalent, to ask that they direct that the council make a decision. This is done through the Planning Inspectorate whose current address is, the Planning Inspectorate, Zone 4/04, Temple Quay House, 2 The Square, Temple Quay, Bristol, BS1 6EB. The application for this will be virtually the same form as your original application for the decision; it is probably easiest to send an entire photocopy of your application together with a covering letter explaining what your application is for. The Countryside Commission and the DEFRA have a useful booklet called *A Guide to Definitive Map Procedures* which you should obtain.

If you think there is any unreasonable delay on the part of the council in processing your application, or they are deliberately going slow, then you could contact the Ombudsman. For information about this contract The Local Government Ombudsman, 21 Queen Anne's Gate, London, SW1H 9BU. The Ombudsman can criticise but doesn't actually have any powers to achieve what you want, which is the decision about the path. Therefore this might prove a lot of work for nothing and might even hold up your original application further while the Ombudsman makes enquiries into the delay. Procedures do take time; try to keep pressure on those obliged to make the decision without making a total nuisance of yourself and without being unrealistic about how long things take.

The Secretary of State for DEFRA can create a new bridleway by statute under the provisions of the Highways Act 1980 section 26 where there is a need for it and it is 'expedient' to create it. This is called making a 'public path order'. There is a formal procedure for this, with time limits where representations and objections can be made. Notice of the making of an order must be placed in local newspapers and given to the local and Parish Councils amongst others. You should therefore keep a close eye on the papers and your Parish Council minutes – even attend the meetings – if you want to hear of this. If you think a bridleway should be created, start by suggesting it to your parish council. A bridleway created like this is maintained at public expense.

As well as challenging path classifications, you could also try to persuade local landowners and/or Parish Councils that new bridleways should be opened by agreement.

If as a landowner you create a horse ride, a cross country course or the like, then remember that it must be safe to use and well maintained, you must have the correct planning permission, you should have investigated whether rates are payable, and insurance cover should be in place. You should also make sure that there is a notice negating the intention to dedicate the ride of track as a right of way, even though it is unlikely that a ride used only on payment of a fee would be classified as a public right of way. If you are trying to achieve more riding space, persuasion based on hard evidence can often be better than unfocused and unrealistic demands.

Upkeep of bridleways

Assuming that you have been successful in an application to the council and on order has been granted, there is now a new bridleway to use. Who is responsible for its upkeep? The Highway Authority must survey the bridleway once the order is made and must specify in a certificate what work is necessary to make it suitable for use as a bridleway. Then the Highway Authority should carry out the work set out in that certificate, although the cost of the work is usually borne by the local authority making the order. Compensation can form part of the cost of the work if, for instance, the landowner loses part of their land.

If someone refuses to maintain a bridleway and it is their responsibility to do so, then the Highways Authority can do the work and recover the cost from the person who should have done the work. The Highways Authority must give that person notice of their intention to do the work and must give them a reasonable opportunity to make the repairs themselves (section 57 of the Highways Act 1980). The duty to repair is to keep the path 'reasonably passable' for its purpose, which would include removing obstacles such as perhaps overhanging trees or encroaching undergrowth, but there is no duty to upgrade the path and make it into a better state than it was originally. Gates, stiles, bridges, etc. have to be kept in a safe condition. The Highways Act 1980, section 146, says that not only should the gates and stiles, etc. be safe, but they must be maintained 'to a standard of repair required to prevent unreasonable interference of the rights of the persons using the footpath or bridleway'. Thus, gates should open, bridges should be wide enough to ride over safely and low branches should be cut back.

Maintenance groups

As a horse rider you could help out by perhaps helping to organise a bridleway maintenance group in your area. Although, technically, maintenance is the duty of the local authorities and landowners, you may find that they never get round to it or don't have the finances to devote to bridleways, which may be fairly low on the local authority's priorities. Therefore, as a matter of practicality, it may well be just as easy to do it yourself. You will find that you need the permission of the owner/ occupier of the land on which the bridleway is situated, and from your local Parish Council and/or the highway authority. Try to get volunteers well in advance as you will always need more people than you think. You will need proper tools for doing the job, but do be careful if you are using machinery. Mechanical tools should only be used by those qualified to do so and everyone else should keep out of the way. The size of the project will dictate the amount of organisation needed. If all you are doing is trimming back a hedge on a short length of bridleway, then it may need no more than half a dozen people with shears and secateurs willing to give up an afternoon. If, on the other hand, major clearance work is required, then clearly much more organisation and time will be required.

Do work closely with the landowner at all times. Establish whether all the rubbish is to be carried away to local tips or whether it can be burnt or put through a compost machine on site; and do, as usual, take out insurance cover. The British Horse Society provide free legal liability insurance cover to any working party clearing bridleways, provided the working party is organised by members of the British Horse Society or by an affiliated bridleways association, and provided the British Horse Society is aware of the working party through notice of it being given to the British Horse Society County Access and Bridleways Officer for the area.

Make sure that you know exactly the extent to which you can clear the bridleway and do not go beyond that. You may find that in some cases the Parish Council would be willing to contribute to the upkeep of bridleways, so it may be worth applying to them particularly if the bridleway is used by a significant proportion of the population in that area.

Signposts

Where a bridleway leaves a metal road, the highway authority must erect and maintain a signpost indicating that there is a bridleway and indicating where it leads and how far away that place is. Obviously the local authority needs the permission of the landowner to put up the signpost and should consult with them first. Signposts need not be erected if it is not thought to be necessary, but should be put up if required to assist people unfamiliar with the area to follow the path or bridleway. Consultation with the Parish Council will be needed to decide on what is necessary. Therefore, representations should be made to your Parish Council if you think clearer signposting is necessary on bridleways. A landowner could put up his or her own signs if the highway authority gives consent. It is suggested that a lot of problems could be overcome with the provision of more signposts and direction signs. Too often, a path can appear to come to a full stop or can end at a field or T-junction, and it is unclear where to go next. Riders are then left with a choice of hoping for the best and going forward, risking the wrath of the landowner if they have gone the wrong way, or turning round and heading back the way they have come. The signs need only be small but clear directional arrows certainly would be welcomed by riders; riders are usually anxious to stay on the correct path and do not wish to cause any damage or ride where they shouldn't.

If you are a landowner, you must not put up a sign at or near a legal path which might suggest riders are prohibited, or which might serve to deter people from using the path. This is a criminal offence punishable by a fine and an order to remove the notice.

As a rider, if in doubt as to where you can ride, check with the Parish Council, the local highway authority or the definitive map which is available for inspection to find out where bridleways or other permitted rides are.

Ploughing

A further problem is ploughing. It is legal for farmers and landowners to plough up bridleways, but it must be necessary to do this within the rules of 'good husbandry' and it must be inconvenient to avoid the bridleway. However, where this has happened, the path must be put back within certain time limits. Rights of way around headlands should not be disturbed at all.

Cycle tracks and bridleways

The Cycle Tracks Act 1984 allows conversion of footpaths into highways that can be used by both walkers and cyclists, but section 26 of the Highways Act 1980 can be used instead. Under this, an order can be given allowing riders access as well. Cyclists can use bridleways, whereas riders cannot always use cycle roads, either by law or because the surface is not suitable – it might be tarmac allowing only walking or some trotting. If your local authority is considering a new cycle path, you could lobby it to consider making a track suitable for both riders and cyclists. This can be done by the use of different surfaces – turf or beaten earth for the riders with a hard surface by the side for cyclists. It may not be ideal, but better than nothing. Cyclists must give way to walkers and riders on bridleways.

It is always better to put proposals for facilities for horses to authorities *before* structures and roads are built, because it is much easier to incorporate facilities into development than to add them afterwards. This is particularly noticeable on major road developments or new housing and village developments. You could campaign for proper and safe bridges over motorways or busy roads to connect existing bridleway networks, or for horse crossing points and underpasses, etc.

There are certain standards to which such structures should conform. As an example, bridleway bridges should be at least 2.7 m wide with parapets high enough to prevent horses being frightened by the sight of traffic below. The surfacing should not, for instance, be steel or aluminium as this would be slippery and noisy and likely to cause accidents. Such features can easily be incorporated into developments at little cost at the planning and building stage, but are likely to be expensive and difficult to incorporate later so are unlikely to be done, with a resulting loss of bridleways and connections.

The British Horse Society have many informative leaflets with regard to bridleways and rights of way and it is well worth obtaining them. They are free, but the Society request that you enclose a stamped addressed envelope.

Dealing with obstructions

Bridleways must remain 'open'. This means that there should be no locked gates, impassable stiles, cattle grids, etc. Cattle grids can only be constructed on highways which have vehicular rights and even then, the cattle grid must allow for other traffic, including ridden horses and horses and carriages, to pass over them. If a route is continually blocked, whether deliberately or not, then it is possible to get an injunction against the landowner causing the obstruction, but of course this will not make you very popular in the neighbourhood. Negotiation with the landowner or other person responsible should be the first step, if it is possible to identify the landowner. If you think negotiation is not a possibility or you don't know who the landowner is, then the highway authority have authority to remove obstructions if requested to do so. As a last resort, a person obstructing the right of way can be prosecuted under section 137 of the Highways Act 1980, but again, this could cause resentment against you and all local riders in the neighbourhood. Sometimes however it may prove necessary where an individual is being deliberately and consistently obstructive. The threat of action might be enough to make them give in, or alternatively you could consider discussing diversion of the path or an alternative path.

Animals on or near bridleways

Dogs

Do be careful if you like to take your dog out riding with you. All dogs in public places should have a name tag showing the owner's name and address.

If your dog attacks 'livestock', which is defined under section 11 of the Animals Act 1971 and includes not only sheep but also cattle, horses and domestic fowl, and pheasants, partridges and grouse in captivity, you could find yourself liable for any injury caused, under section 3 of the same Act. Again, as with all Animals Act cases, not only the owner of the dog could be liable but also the 'keeper' of it. Where the rider with the dog is under 16 years old, liability could rest with the head of the household.

You could also find yourself liable under the Dogs (Protection of Livestock) Act 1953 if the dog worries livestock on *agricultural* land. Agricultural land is generally meadow or grazing land, but the definition also includes such areas as allotments under section 3 of the Act. There are defences available under the Act, for example, you can seek to prove that when the dog attacked the livestock it was not you that was in control of the dog, but someone else who you reasonably believed was a proper person to be in charge of it. Under the Act, the police can impound a dog where the owner cannot be found. If you have to go to the police station to get the dog released, not only might you be charged with an offence, but you will also have to pay the expenses incurred by the police in keeping the dog until you came forward.

Sheep are particularly protected as it is an offence to allow a dog to be loose in a field or on land where there are sheep; it must be on a lead or under 'close control'. There are exemptions, such as packs of hounds and police dogs. We all believe that our dogs are beautifully trained and could be said to be under close control, but any dog can lose its head in the excitement of the moment and the best advice has to be to keep your dog on a lead at all times. However, do remember that it is not safe to ride while leading a dog – you could easily be pulled from the saddle by a dog taking off after a rabbit or other livestock.

Under section 8 of the Animals Act 1971, as the owner or keeper of a dog, you have a duty to take reasonable care that damage is not caused by your dog straying onto the highway. If your dog is involved in a road accident as a result of which it is injured, the driver must stop. This is the same if there is an accident with horses. The purpose of the driver being required to stop is so that names, addresses and registration numbers of the vehicles can be exchanged. If this is not possible then the accident must be reported to a police station as soon as reasonably practicable and in any case within 24 hours of the accident (Road Traffic Act 1922 section 25).

You can also be liable if your dog attacks another person, particularly if you know they are inclined to do that.

Ultimately, your dog could be legally killed under section 9 of the Animals Act 1971. It is a defence under this Act to show that the dog was killed or injured, usually by shooting, while it was worrying or about to worry animals and there was no other reasonable means of stopping or preventing the worrying, or that the dog had been worrying animals and was still roaming free under no obvious control and there appeared no means of finding out to whom it belonged.

Usually the only person entitled to shoot the dog to protect animals is the owner of the animals, or the owner or occupier of the land on which the animals are being worried, or someone authorised by them. Therefore, for instance, a shepherd employed by the owner of the land could legally shoot a dog worrying his sheep. If a dog is shot or injured in this way, then notice must be given to an 'officer in charge of a police station' within 48 hours of the death or injury.

You cannot shoot a dog worrying animals where the animals have escaped onto someone else's land and the dog doing the worrying belongs to the owner or occupier of the land onto which they have strayed.

If offences involving dogs can be shown, liability for injury done by dogs to animals is 'strict'. That means that it is enough to show that the injury or death of the animal has been caused by the dog; there is no need to prove that the owner or keeper of the dog was negligent in allowing it to do so. You can also be liable for damage done to land or property by your dog. If your dog strays onto land, the owner of the land can keep the dog until you claim it and you will be liable for expenses incurred while keeping it, such as feeding it.

From the alternative perspective, riders do have a right to expect that they can ride along legal bridleways and other roads without being unduly harassed or worried by animals. So if you are walking your dog do keep it on a lead if you know that there are likely to be horses about, or at the very least make sure that it is trained well enough to come to call and sit quietly by you while horses pass.

One of the most annoying things for a rider is dogs jumping up and barking behind fencing which adjoins a bridle path or other road.

Unfortunately, this does not appear to constitute a nuisance or obstruction. In the case of *Kent County Council* v. *Holland* (1996) (Horse Law (1997) Vol. 2, Iss. 1), a complaint was made under s137 of the Highways Act. It was alleged that dogs leaping up at a fence and barking at people constituted an obstruction because their presence 'instilled fear in the users of the pathway'. It was held that the dogs might well be a nuisance, but were not an obstruction. An action for nuisance was not however, guaranteed to succeed and was likely to be expensive. There is very little that can be done about it other than avoiding the dog or that path if you know your horse is going to be bothered by it.

Bird scarers

Bird scarers on or near a public path or ride can also cause problems. It is not illegal to have a bird scarer near a path, but if the landowner knew that horses use the path and that the bird scarer going off at intervals would be likely to cause horses to take fright, then if a rider was injured when this happened, the landowner might be liable under the general law of negligence.

Bulls

Bulls should not generally be kept in fields which have a right of way through them, but under section 59 of the Wildlife and Countryside Act 1981 a bull can be kept in a field if it is less than ten months old or is not one of the dairy breeds and is running with cows or heifers. Even though this may be legal, it can still be quite a frightening experience and there is no guarantee that the bulls and cows will not, out of curiosity if nothing else, crowd round you or charge up to your horse and frighten it. Are you confident you can tell the difference between a ten month old bull and a twelve month old bull? Can you even remember which are dairy breeds and which are beef breeds?

If this situation is a constant problem, even where allowed under section 59, you could look at whether the action of the animals comes under section 2 of the Animals Act 1971, which provides that a keeper of an animal is liable for damage caused by an animal not belonging to a dangerous species if the animal has a particular characteristic over and above any 'normally' dangerous characteristic of that type of animal. The text of section 2 was set out in Chapter 2, in the section on injury caused by animals.

To put this into the context of bulls, imagine the bull was a beef breed such as a Hereford and was therefore legally in the field. Bulls might have a 'normal' characteristic of charging. However, if this particular bull was known by its owner to be especially likely to, say, charge trotting horses, then there might possibly be liability if it did then charge at you causing injury while you were trotting through its field. In the context of horses, say, for instance, you normally ride through a field where there are mares who are usually quiet, but are known to be vicious if they have foals at foot. It might be wise for the owner either to turn the mares out into another field where there is no right of way or to fence them off.

In the case of *Miller* v. *Duggan*, heard in Warrington County Court in 1996, Mr Miller, the claimant, was walking his dog along a public footpath where horses owned by the defendant were grazing. Apparently the horses gathered around him and pushed him to the ground, causing injury. Mr Miller alleged it was negligent of the defendant to graze horses where he knew people were going to be walking. His claim was dismissed. There was no evidence that this had happened before, nor that the horses were dangerous; they were just acting as horses do. It may be unreasonable to suggest that horses never be grazed anywhere people are likely to be where there is no particular perceived risk from the horses.

As a practical solution, polite requests to put some sort of fencing along the right of way to separate the animals from the horse riders might work. It might be worth asking the Parish Council whether they would be willing to pay for this, particularly if you could get a group of local people to provide the labour for free. While a farmer might argue that it is his field and he can do what he likes with it, he might be wise to weigh up the cost of fencing as against a potential claim running into millions of pounds if someone is severely injured or dies as a result of an incident.

Trespass

Obviously, riders should not trespass onto land and most, if not all, riders will take the utmost care not to do so. Good signposting, as mentioned earlier, can help. A misleading sign is the 'Trespassers will be prosecuted' notice. You cannot be prosecuted i.e. held liable under criminal law, just for a trespass, but if you do cause damage you could be prosecuted and liable to the landowner for compensation for that damage.

You will no doubt be pleased to know that if your horse gets out of control and runs away with you, then the law has some sympathy and will not add to your troubles by making you liable for a trespass in those circumstances, even where you go onto someone else's land. You have to *intend* to go onto someone else's land where you should not be, but even an unintentional wandering onto someone else's property can be a trespass. Once you find you are trespassing, you should leave the land as soon as possible by the shortest way you can, but without doing any damage.

If you are the landowner and you find someone trespassing, you should first ask the horse and rider to leave the land. You will find that most riders, once it is made known to them that they are trespassing, will be only too glad to go back to where they should be. If the trespasser refuses to leave, then reasonable force can be used to make them leave, but the question of what is 'reasonable force' is open to any amount of legal argument. It is important that reasonable force does not slip over into unnecessary force, as then the person using the unnecessary force may be liable for assault. There are numerous cases concerning hunts where hunt servants or followers have been found liable or have been prosecuted for assault where they are trying to remove hunt protesters from land. Where cases have succeeded, many have been overturned but not without the necessity and expense, to say nothing of the trauma, of going to appeal.

If during a hunt, the hunt servants or field trespass, then the master of hounds may be liable for their trespass, as well as the servants and field members themselves. The master will be liable for trespass by hounds if he allows hounds to hunt somewhere that he knows gives no option but to trespass or if he knows there is a risk that they will do so, or if he fails to prevent trespass due to negligence, i.e. in failing to have the pack under proper control.

Footpaths are for 'passing and re-passing'. Therefore, if you stand still on a footpath for a considerable length of time, say during a protest, you may be held to be causing an obstruction and thus likely to be causing an offence and removed and/or prosecuted. Trying to get round this by constantly moving up and down the same short stretch of path can also be obstruction.

It is not a good idea to try to establish a right of way or a bridleway by continually trespassing over land in the hope that the landowner will eventually give in. It will almost certainly have the opposite effect and you, as a rider, could find yourself on the receiving end of an injunction stopping you riding there, and you will certainly spoil the chances of other riders ever establishing good relationships with the landowner that might have led to them being allowed to use the land.

Chapter 12
Trailers and Horseboxes

We have all seen the monster 10 or 12 horseboxes used by race horse transporters or professional riders, but many amateur riders now have a trailer or small horsebox.

Trailers

Insurance

Your normal car insurance should cover you to tow a trailer as long as the trailer is within permitted weight ratios, whether it is your own trailer or someone else's, but it will not cover you if you are paying that person a commercial rate to loan their trailer, or they are loaning the trailer for hire or reward. It is all right to borrow a friend's trailer and perhaps buy them a box of chocolates or fill their lorry up with petrol as a thank you, but you may not be covered for anything more commercial than that. Your basic car insurance may only cover you for accidents which happen while you are towing and is unlikely to cover damage to the trailer itself or damage caused solely by the trailer. If you want cover to include the trailer itself you will need a separate trailer insurance to cover damage to and by the trailer, or fire and theft to the trailer itself. Otherwise you may find that the trailer is not separately insured and is not protected while unhitched from the car. Check the terms of the separate insurance as many policies will want the trailer locked when not attached to the vehicle or kept inside a locked building when parked. You may also find that your trailer insurance does not cover you for third party liability – that is, damage or injury caused to a third party by the trailer itself, rather than the trailer being damaged, lost or stolen. This might be covered under your car insurance, but do check.

It is difficult, if not impossible, to find an insurer who will insure your towing vehicle and a trailer as a complete package. Usually you will find these have to be insured separately. It is well worth taking out an insurance that includes a recovery service and provision of a vet if needed, or the use of alternative transport of overnight stabling and accommodation. A number of specialist insurers advertise at the back of horse magazines. There is also an organisation called the Organisation of Horse Box and Trailer Owners who provide various services to owners, including an insurance service.

Driving tests

Drivers who passed their test prior to 1 January 1997 can drive trailers and some other classes of vehicle but it is advisable to undertake a trailer driving course, or at the very least to practise on some open ground away from public roads, before venturing out and particularly before venturing out fully loaded. If, however, you passed your test after 1 January 1997 then you may need to take a further test or tests before you can tow a trailer or other horseboxes. You can tow with L-plates under the supervision of a person qualified to tow. You should contact the National Trailer and Towing Association or the Driving and Vehicle Licensing Agency in Swansea for full details. For how to take tests, contact your local driving test centre. The National Trailer and Towing Association provide residential courses with the test taken at the end. They can also send instructors out where there are a number of people in the same area requiring tuition, but the test cannot be taken in these circumstances. Trailer manufacturers Ifor Williams show some training and test providers on their website. The test will include meeting certain medical and eyesight standards, reversing off and on road, emergency stops and driving in the city as well as country, perhaps even on a motorway where possible. You will also need to be able to competently hitch up and unhitch a trailer.

The British Horse Society produces and sells a booklet *Towing and Trailers*, part of which is reproduced in Appendix 4 of this book, giving details of when you will need further tests and what you can legally drive. For more information about almost anything to do with towing, towing vehicles, trailers and horseboxes, look out for books and articles by John Henderson, who writes extensively on the subject, or contact the National Trailer and Towing Association.

Size of trailer

If the towing vehicle exceeds 3.5 tonnes gross then the trailer to be towed cannot exceed 12 m long and 2.55 m wide. If the towing vehicle is under 3.5 tonnes then the restrictions are 7 m long and 2.3 m wide. The overall length of the towing vehicle and trailer combined must not exceed 18 m.

The recommended guideline for maximum height is 3 m, or 1.7 times the wheel track, which is the horizontal distance between the centre lines of tyre treads, although there is no legal requirement for this. Check carefully that your towing vehicle can legally tow your trailer from a weight point of view. Calculating the legal weights can be a complicated business – there are kerb weights, maximum gross weights, maximum permissible weights, gross train weights, maximum authorised masses – and it can get confusing. Rather than try to work it out yourself, contact the organisations referred to above, with the make and model of the towing vehicle and trailer – preferably before you make a purchase – to check if they are compatible and legal. Trailer and towing vehicle dealers and manufacturers should be able to help and your car and trailer handbooks will give details of weights. There are differences for braked and unbraked trailers.

When calculating the laden weight of the trailer remember to include the weight of saddles, tack, harness, hay nets and the general clutter that you transport around, as well as of your horse or horses. Consider whether a single horse trailer would suit your needs, as this would weigh less.

Safety

There is no mandatory requirement for a trailer to have an annual MOT test, nor are they plated like lorries, but this does not mean that you can avoid maintaining the trailer. If you are involved in an accident and the cause of the accident is the fact that you haven't maintained your trailer – say, for instance, the brakes are defective – then it is no excuse to say that there is no law to say that the trailer has to be serviced. You would still be negligent and probably liable for the damage and injury caused and for compensation. It is particularly important to check over and service both trailers and horseboxes once they have been standing for a time, such as during the winter. At the very least you should check all the things you would check on a car, such as tyres, brakes, lights, etc., and in particular you should keep a careful eye on the flooring of your trailer. Many trailers have a wooden flooring, which can rot; a number of manufacturers will replace wooden flooring with aluminium flooring at a reasonable cost. Trailers must carry a plate with the registration number of the towing vehicle on it. Do not forget to change the trailer registration plate if you change the towing vehicle – this is easily overlooked.

If you loan your trailer to someone and their horse is injured because you have neglected to maintain your trailer – for instance, it might have some sharp edges sticking out or have unsafe or slippery flooring on the ramp – you could possibly be liable. While it is neighbourly to loan out your trailer to those who have no transport, be very careful about doing so.

You should not travel in a trailer with your horses, although you can travel in the living area of a horsebox. Bear in mind that there are unlikely to be any safety belts in this living area so if there is an accident there is more potential for injury than if you are travelling in the towing vehicle or the front of the horsebox.

Lorries

Tests on lorries and trailers

If you are buying a lorry, do check that the numbers on the plate and on the lorry itself match up. There will also be numbers in the lorry's engine and on its chassis which should match. If they do not, it may be an indication that it has been stolen, with the body of the stolen box having been transferred onto a different chassis, although professionals will almost certainly have altered the numbers to match. They might also have made alterations to the body, such as putting in windows or repainting it, although of course there are genuine sellers who make attempts to smarten up their box before selling it. If you are buying a horsebox conversion, usually you will be buying a new body on a lorry chassis. You may want to consider etching the engine and chassis numbers on the body, so that all the parts can be matched up, although it is a relatively simple job to alter these if someone is intent on being dishonest.

Lorries have to be tested annually to ensure that they are roadworthy, in much the same way that a car is given an annual MOT test. It is known as 'plating' because once a lorry has been satisfactorily tested a plate or certificate is placed in the cab of the lorry. Plating applies to lorries where the chassis is more than three years old. Do remember that you still have to maintain the lorry properly between platings. The fact that a lorry has a valid plate does not mean that it is roadworthy; it will still need regular checks and servicing.

Horseboxes

Buying a horsebox can be almost as trying as buying the horse itself. You should always take someone experienced with you when buying a box, or buy from a specialist dealer who may well offer a warranty. You can have a 'provenance check' carried out. Companies such as South Essex Insurance Brokers can do these. They trace the history of the box so that you can ensure it is legitimate. There is a small fee for this but it is well worth doing, and some insurers who carry out the service will refund the cost of it if you then insure with them. At the time of writing, provenance checks can also be done by the AA or the RAC, if you are a member. If you do it through the AA, then if the AA provides incorrect information, it does have a compensation scheme.

Tachographs

From 1 April 2002, all horseboxes fitted with a tachograph will have the tachograph checked annually. This applies even to privately owned boxes which aren't normally subject to the same tachograph regulations as commercial users. Commercial use can be interpreted quite strictly. If there is any element of hire or reward in the use of a horsebox or trailer, then a tachograph may not only need to be fitted, but actually in use. If, for instance, you have a small stud and are driving your own horses to a show where there is the possibility of winning prize money, this could be interpreted as a reward.

A tachograph is checked when first installed in a lorry, to see that it is recording mileage correctly, and a seal is put on it. This seal will be checked at each plating. When buying a lorry, check to see that the seal has not been tampered with. You can telephone the Vehicle Inspectorate on 0870 6060 440 for an information leaflet on tachographs.

Security

As an extra security feature, you might want to paint your registration number on top of your box or trailer, and also possibly install an alarm, an immobiliser or even a tracking device which sends out signals enabling the trailer or box to be tracked if it is stolen. If you have these extras, you may find that your insurance premium is reduced.

Chapter 13
Safety at Shows and Other Events

If you are the organiser of an event or show, you will have a duty of care to those taking part, both spectators and competitors. Competitors will be assumed in most cases to accept the risks inherent and foreseeable in the sport itself. Thus, as the organiser, you may not be liable if a horse falls at a fence throwing off its rider and injuring him or her. That would be a foreseeable risk of the sport as everyone knows that from time to time horses fall and riders fall off. On the other hand, you may be liable if the reason the horse fell was because you had failed to notice and eradicate a huge rabbit hole which the horse put its foot down, causing it to fall. This is not a risk of the sport as such, even though it is a foreseeable accident. It is a risk which could be guarded against or eradicated altogether. The rider is deemed to know there is a risk of a fall and to accept that risk, but would not be deemed to accept the risk of a fall due to someone else's negligence.

Competitors have a duty of care to spectators, who are deemed to accept a certain amount of risk themselves as spectators. For instance, at a three-day event, despite the precautions of the riders and the organisers in setting ride boundaries and fences to keep spectators away from the course, the collecting ring, etc., sometimes an accident will happen. A horse might go out of control after a fall and try and jump a boundary fence, landing among spectators and causing injury. This may turn out to be 'just one of those things' and not negligent, and therefore no claim can follow. If on the other hand a rider is riding a clearly unsuitable horse which they cannot control and the reason it falls is because the rider is clearly being run away with, then this might be said to be negligent as the rider should have known better. You would also have to look at how far the organisers of the show had control over the standard of entry.

Organisers should ensure that spectators cannot get too close to the action. If a spectator is injured due to wandering off permitted areas onto the course or into the ring, then it may be their own fault and they may even be liable themselves if someone, for instance a rider, is injured due to colliding with them or trying to avoid them. A spectator may try to argue that they were not sure where they were allowed to go and where they were not allowed to go because the signs were unclear. As an organiser, make sure that no-go areas are very clearly signposted and roped or railed off. Remember that some of your spectators will be children and there may be some people who cannot read too well due to poor eyesight, so make sure that your signs are large and noticeable and not obscured.

As an organiser, you can be liable under the Occupiers' Liability Act 1957 for injuries caused by your negligence to certain categories of people. Under this Act, you have a duty of care to anyone who might reasonably be expected to be on the land or premises that you are 'occupying'. You cannot escape liability as an organiser by saying that you do not own the land or premises and that you are only using, renting, or borrowing them for a particular purpose for a short time. You can be an occupier for a very short time but it is down to you to make the land and premises safe for the period that you are occupying them. It doesn't matter that the farmer who owns the land hasn't bothered to fill in rabbit holes; it will be your duty to do so if necessary.

Risk assessment

If you are running a show or event you will need to carry out a risk assessment beforehand and take steps to eliminate or at least reduce the identified risks as far as possible. Each event will have its own risks and there is no sure way of identifying every one. As long as you have done your best, credit will be given, even if it does not enable you to escape liability altogether. An absence of a risk assessment could be taken as evidence that you didn't even begin to think about safety. As a rule of thumb, if you think something might be dangerous or cause an accident, it probably is and will. It doesn't matter if an accident happens in a way you didn't envisage; it is enough to be able to see that an accident of some sort might occur.

You can bring in health and safety consultants to carry out risk assessments, or you can do them yourself. You will have to weigh up the cost of this in relation to the nature and size of your event and the likely consequences of any risk materialising. If, for instance, your livery yard is hosting a very small dressage competition for local riders using only your own arena, with not more than about 15 people, it is probably not worthwhile to have a professional assessment carried out. You just need to do your own risk assessment, assuming your premises are relatively safe already.

On the other hand if you are organising a pony club rally or a riding club camp with many different horses and riders, particularly children at a strange venue, then you may wish to err on the side of caution and get a professional assessment done. You may have a higher duty of care to children than to adults. If you need convincing, weigh up the cost of having a risk assessment done as against what you might have to pay if there is a very serious accident, and decide whether you can afford to take the risk. You could perhaps pay for one professional assessment and comply with that, and then use it as a basis for future risk assessments carried out by yourself, provided there were no major changes to the venue or event.

Do make sure that you are insured, but also check your policy carefully and check with your insurance company as your insurance could be invalidated if you have not taken all reasonable precautions to make your event safe. This might include having a risk assessment done. Do not assume that all policies are the same, or that if you have a policy from the same insurer it will be the same as the one you had last year.

The following are examples of points to be considered during a risk assessment:

- How are people going to get in and out? Will it be possible to separate traffic, pedestrians and riders, or if not do you need to put staff in place to ensure horseboxes drive slowly and in one direction away from pedestrians, with pedestrians being kept in a different part of a roadway or entrance?
- Can you have a large enough space as a collecting ring so that horses do not barge into each other, particularly if there is a practice jump? In September 2001 *Horse Law* reported the case of *Justin Peter Lloyd* v. *Wembley Stadium* (2001). The claimant, Mr Lloyd, was exercising his horse in an exercise arena prior to competing. Even at 6.30AM, there were approximately 80–100 riders in the exercise arena. Mr Lloyd became concerned for the safety of himself and his horse, considering the arena overcrowded, and he tried to leave. As he did so, his horse was overtaken by another horse which bucked and kicked out as it passed, fracturing Mr Lloyd's right leg. The stadium's defence was that a crowded arena was a common situation at competitions and Mr Lloyd well knew of the potential problems and thus could be said to have accepted the risks. There had been no previous accidents of this nature, apparently. Nevertheless, the stadium was found liable. The judge felt that there should have been some limit on numbers, with enough stewards to enforce the limit. The stadium had not done enough to ensure the arena was safe. Mr Lloyd could not be said to have accepted the risk. He had done all he could by riding when he thought it would be quiet and trying to leave when he felt the situation was becoming unsafe.
- Are there enough helpers to lift heavy objects such as jump poles or

wings so that no one gets hurt lifting? You may need to check whether your event is covered by the Manual Handling Regulations 1995 (Statutory Instrument 1992 No. 2793), which govern lifting, carrying, moving weighty items and use of lifting equipment. They apply to employers, but the regulations themselves give useful information and advice on lifting and avoiding injury and are worth looking at even in a non-employment context.

- Are there any overhanging trees or cables? Can the branches be cut down or can the event rings or parking be sited well away from any cables?
- What is the ground like? Does it need rolling? Is it very slippery? Do you need to sand the jumping track? Is the take-off and landing area likely to become poached and dangerous? Make a last check on the actual day of the event and if it is bad weather keep checking. Your insurance may cover you for cancellation for bad weather, but only if you call off an event or class before a certain time.
- Are there enough people to act as stewards to ensure safety? Ensure all stewards and officials, fence judges, etc. are equipped with the means to warn people of dangers, e.g. approaching horses. Most people will react to a sharp whistle blast.
- Do you have safe fencing to keep spectators away from a course or a ring? Consider what type of fencing to use. Sometimes this can be difficult. Do you have a solid barrier between the spectators and the horses, which may deter horses from running into it but which may fool them into thinking it is a jump; or do you have ropes which may give way in an emergency but would not stop a crush of spectators being pushed forward onto a course if there are a lot of people? It may not matter which, as long as you can show that you have given thought to the matter and that your choice is reasonable for the cir-cumstances. The main point is to keep spectators off the course, not horses and riders on it.

Wooldridge v. *Sumner* ((1962) 2 All ER 978, (1963) 2 QB 43) is one of the leading cases on spectators and sport. In this case, a hunter was being shown in the galloping phase of the show class at White City in 1959. The horse cornered too fast and collided with and injured a cameraman at the edge of the ring. Interestingly, the cameraman was injured when he was trying to pull a lady spectator out of the way of the horse, which he feared would injure her. He had been sitting on a bench and had he continued to do so, the likelihood was that he would not have been injured.

The cameraman sued the rider, together with the British Horse Society as the show organisers and 'occupiers' at that time, but the case against the BHS was dismissed.

The claimant, the cameraman, initially won his case, but then lost it on appeal. The court found that the rider had not been negligent. The horse was being deliberately ridden at a fast speed, as required by the competition, but was under sufficient control all the time. The rider might have made an error of judgement, but that did not constitute negligence. It appears that courts realise that spectators do have to accept a certain level of risk when attending a sporting event, and that risk is that riders may make such errors of judgement or suffer 'lapses of skill' momentarily. However, it is unlikely that spectators would be taken to have accepted the risk of a rider being reckless for their own or other's safety, or deliberately riding dangerously, if an injury were to follow as a result.

- Is your course safe? Consider whether a riders' advocate should be appointed to raise safety issues with the organiser, e.g. is a fence too difficult or too much of a 'trap' for the standard of entry. This is not to say that courses should be kept artificially simple, but sometimes they may be just too difficult for expected standards of competition. The identity of the rider advocate for each event should be clearly posted and made known to competitors.
- The mobile telephone, while being a nuisance in some ways, is an essential tool now for health and safety should the emergency services need to be called. Make sure all stewards are in contact with a central point either by telephone or radio link. Ensure they can all give a description of their location. Have all essential names, addresses and telephone numbers in a prominent place with a copy given to all helpers. Have fire extinguishers and other precautions available and ensure everyone knows how to use them.
- Do not let children or untrained or inexperienced people use quad bikes or other all terrain vehicles, however much fun it is tearing round a showground. Those who do use them should have or be provided with a suitable protective helmet. If they are to go on a public road at all, the vehicles must have proper insurance. Accidents which occur if these vehicles are on a public road may come under the vehicles' own insurance and not any public liability insurance taken out for the event. You can hire teams of quad bikes and riders who are likely to have their own insurance.
- Dogs must be on leads.

This is not a definitive list, just some thoughts on the type of thing to look out for. The British Horse Society produce a leaflet *Health and Safety Guidelines* which is very useful.

The higher the risk, the greater the need for safety. Look at what level of injury could occur if the risk was not eradicated or reduced, i.e. is something so dangerous that it could lead to death or serious injury, such as an electric cable being within touching distance, or is it merely an inconvenience? You must look at how likely the risk is to materialise and cause an injury. You must take all reasonable and practicable measures in avoiding risks.

Medical cover

Ensure that you have adequate medical cover. What is adequate has to be a matter of judgement. At the very least, you will need one or more qualified first-aiders to deal with minor injuries, and a St John's Ambulance team, but this may not be sufficient. If the likelihood of serious injury is high, a St John's Ambulance team may not be deemed adequate. You might need a qualified doctor, a paramedic team and medical equipment on hand to give emergency treatment, and even access to an air ambulance in some cases. From a medic's point of view, if you are asked to officiate as a doctor at an event, do consider whether your expertise is sufficient for you to do the job properly. You may be a superb gynaecologist, but would you feel confident in dealing with what looks like a possible severe brain injury or cardiac arrest in less than ideal conditions? There is a qualification in pre-hospital or advanced trauma life support for NHS qualified people, such as nurses or doctors, that teaches what to do in the immediate aftermath of an accident or other trauma.

With some injuries, such as spinal or head injuries, appropriate and immediate treatment can make all the difference between a person becoming seriously disabled or even dying, and a full or near full recovery. If a delay in getting proper treatment has been the cause of somebody's injury or even death, it could be negligent if you did not have appropriate medical care there. The Medical Equestrian Association highlights areas where safety could be improved and campaigns for better care at equestrian events.

There is no duty on other riders or spectators to assist where they see an accident or someone suffering an illness, but if you do go to help – it is almost a reflex to do so – then make sure you only go if and when it is safe to do so. There is no point dashing to someone's aid only to be trampled by the next oncoming horse, causing further injuries. Do not do anything which is likely to make the situation worse, for instance, it is not always a good idea to take off a hat or body protector or move someone. On the other hand, if you can see that someone is very clearly turning blue and choking on their tongue, and you are the only person there, it would probably be appropriate for you to try and relieve this. As a non-medically qualified person, often the best you can do is call for help and keep the area clear for easy access for the medical services.

Keep an accident report book and fill in an accident report form as soon as possible after the accident with as much information as you can. The accident might need to be reported as an incident under the Reporting of Injuries, Diseases and Dangerous Occurrences Regulations 1995 (RID-DOR). Under these regulations, certain accidents or incidents that could have caused an accident are reportable to the Health and Safety Executive. There is a central reporting unit (details are given under 'Useful Addresses'). Briefly, employers have a duty to report deaths or major injuries, work related diseases, accidents at work which cause an employee or self-employed person to be off work for over three days, and 'dangerous occurrences' which could have caused a reportable incident, but didn't. In the context of shows, competitions, rallies, etc, if someone *employed* – either on behalf of the organisers of the event or there in the course of their employment, i.e. a groom – is killed, injured or is subject to a dangerous occurrence, then the matter should be reported by the employer. Incidents occurring to competitors, spectators, etc. *not* there in any employment capacity are not legally required to be reported, but it can be helpful to report them anyway for statistical purposes. Major injuries can include fractures and dislocations, electric shocks leading to unconsciousness, injuries causing loss of consciousness or requiring resuscitation or acute illnesses requiring medical treatment. 'Dangerous occurrences' are set out in Schedule 2 of the Regulations; probably the most relevant in this context is the collapse of a structure, i.e. a grandstand, or incident involving lifting machinery.

You will also need a vet and farrier, if not actually at the event then at least on call and within easy reach.

Liability for injuries

You cannot escape liability by putting up a notice saying that you or the organisation responsible for the show or rally will not be liable for any injuries howsoever caused. This is rendered void by the Unfair Contract Terms Act 1977. If injury or death is caused by the organiser's negligence and can be proved to be so, then the organisers will be liable notwithstanding the notice. It might be worth drawing attention to the fact that you can disclaim other sorts of liability, e.g. loss of or damage to equipment, and that riders do ride at their own risk, but you cannot avoid liability for death or injury that is your fault.

If you do wish to try and rely on a disclaimer to avoid liability, then the notice must be worded in easily understandable plain English and should be prominently displayed, for instance, by a large poster at all entrances to a competition or showground, in car parks and clearly displayed on the *front* of admission tickets and competition entry forms. There is no set wording as long as it is clear to the public that you and/or the organisers are warning them that you will not be responsible for any of their losses, damage or injuries unless it can be shown to be legally your fault. When a member of the public buys a ticket to enter into a competition, they are entering into a contract with the organisers of the show. The disclaimer must be part of that contract; a term of it and to make it so, the term has to be clearly brought to the attention of the buyer before or at the time of making the contract. It may not be part of the contract and therefore cannot be relied on, if it is only brought to someone's attention after they have gone into the show, or after they have bought their ticket.

Two cases are worth looking at. First, in the matter of Rebecca Ward (Deceased) in 1999, an inquest was held at the coroner's court for Spilsby, Lincolnshire (*Horse Law* (1999) Vol. 4, Iss. 4). Miss Ward, aged 14, was at a Pony Club camp. She had been riding since she was about six years old and at the time was riding her own horse, which she had apparently had for about six weeks. While jumping, the horse slipped suddenly, threw Miss Ward and then somersaulted over the fence landing on her and crushing her. Sadly she was killed. She was wearing a hat and body protector and it was thought that but for the horse rolling on her, she might well have been uninjured or at least have survived.

The coroner held that it was an accidental death. It was no fault of the organiser of the camp. The fence was well within the rider's capabilities and was a properly built fence of no particular difficulty. The outcome might have been different if Miss Ward had been urged to jump a fence clearly outside her own or the horse's capability by an instructor engaged by the organisers, or if the fence had been the cause of her death due to being improperly constructed.

In another coroner's decision (Re: Rebecca Nordell (Deceased) (1997) *Horse and Hound* (1998) 15 August, *Horse Law* (1998) Vol. 3, Iss. 6), a horse with a habit of breaking free (although this may have been unknown to the person in charge of the horse at the time of the show) was tied to a piece of baler twine apparently attached to a sheep hurdle outside its horsebox. The horse broke free and bolted around the horsebox area, dragging the hurdle with it. The hurdle struck an 8 year old girl who died later of head injuries.

The coroner found it was unclear whether the person in charge of the horse had tied it to the twine, or to the actual hurdle, with a suggestion that it was in fact tied directly to the hurdle, which may well have been negligent. It is not the function of a coroner's inquest to decide whether someone has or has not been negligent; that is ultimately a matter for the civil courts. The coroner voiced concern about the organisation of the show, and the lack of provision in rural hospitals for the treatment of head injuries – not the organiser's fault of course. The person in charge of the horse was being sued by the deceased girl's parents. It is suggested that the organisers may escape liability in this case. They could be expected to provide enough space to tie up horses safely away from the general public, but probably they could not be responsible for owners' short-comings in tying up their own horses. They could not perhaps be expected to go round every box, insisting that every horse was safely secured.

What organisers can do, however, is impose their own rules and con-ditions on shows and refuse to allow riders to compete if they do not adhere to them. For instance, the organisers can say that every rider must wear a proper hat and a body protector if jumping. You can put this on the entry forms and in the programmes and refuse to allow anyone to com-pete who does not adhere to these rules. You can have as many rules and regulations as you like, but do remember that they will have to be sensible and enforceable if anyone is to take any notice of them. Even if they do not stop accidents completely, at least they draw riders' attention to safety and might perhaps make them think twice before doing something foolish which could cause injury to themselves or others.

Chapter 14
Accidents – When Can I Claim?

There has been an enormous growth in interest in riding accidents and safety, not least because of the tragic death of five event riders in a short time between 1999 and 2000. It is often said that riding is a risk sport, which is true, but no more so surely than Formula I motor racing, mountaineering, or even ski-ing. The aim must be to minimise the risk and make riders aware of the risks they face, so they can decide whether they want to take those risks or not.

Fortunately, the law helps riders as it does recognise that the horse is a separate living being with a mind of its own and it is not possible to be in complete control under every circumstance 100% of the time. In the case of *Haines* v. *Weston* (1981) (RTR 90) a horse and rider were in collision with a car after the horse shied into the car's path. The rider claimed against the car driver but the car driver counter-claimed saying that the rider had allowed the horse to go into the path of the car by failing to stop it shying.

At the first hearing, the judge appeared to agree with the car driver. His judgment suggested that all riders know all horses are likely to shy at almost anything at any time, so they should ensure that they are *always* in control. The rider appealed and the Appeal Court judges decided the decision was wrong. The court said the person making the claim must prove negligence against the person they are suing. If there is no negligence on the part of the person against whom a claim is contemplated or made, then there is no case. The court accepted that sometimes horses do something potentially dangerous even when a rider has taken every precaution. It need not necessarily be a dangerous act in itself. If a Shire horse accidentally walks backwards into a car, damage may be caused purely by the effect of something the size and weight of a Shire knocking into it. No-one need be injured and the handler need not have been negligent. Thus if you, as a rider, are contemplating a claim against a driver, a show organiser, a riding school, etc., you must show that they were legally negligent, i.e. failed in some way to take proper care for your safety. This could mean failing to drive at a safe speed, driving too close to you, failing to ensure a safe surface at a show or giving you an unsuitable horse to ride. In the quoted case, the rider was not negligent even though the horse had shied, because to say that a rider must *always* be in control no matter what the circumstances is to put too high a duty on the rider.

Insurance claims

One point to note is that if an accident happens involving your horse, then even if loss, damage or injury is caused by it, if you were not negligent your insurers may refuse to meet any claim. You may feel that the incident was your fault and you may even want to pay for any damage your horse has caused, but if your insurers consider it a pure accident and not your fault, they will neither pay the person who has suffered the damage nor reimburse you if you have paid for any loss or damage. You may feel morally obliged to pay and if the accident involves someone you know, it may cause embarrassment and ill-feeling if no claim is met, but insurers do not act out of sympathy. They will have to consider you to have been negligent before they will decide whether to pay out or not. This is not the insurers being awkward; the law is that only where negligence can be proved and shown to have caused loss or injury does the right to compensation arise. You should not assume that because you are insured there will be an automatic pay-out, and neither should those injured or suffering financial loss due to your actions.

Do check your policy carefully, as many policies will have a clause forbidding you from accepting or trying to accept liability for an accident. Even an apology can sometimes be construed as an admission. It won't necessarily be, nor will it by itself prove that you are at fault, but the insurers may try to invalidate your policy if you appear to have indicated to the other party that the accident was in some way your fault.

Proving a claim

What often surprises people when they try to make a claim, or do make a claim, is the fact that the law in England and Wales requires the person making the claim to prove every part of it. This means that the person who has suffered the injury, damage or loss has to prove to the requirements of the principles of English law that firstly, the accident was someone else's fault, secondly, that it did cause the injuries complained of, and thirdly, that losses or expenses were actually incurred and/or will be incurred because of the accident. The person also has to prove the extent of those losses or expenses. Strictly speaking, anything that cannot be proved cannot be claimed for.

To claimants this can seem very unfair. They are generally the innocent party and have suffered at the hands of someone else. Why should they have to do all the work necessary to show that they have a genuine claim? Why don't the insurers just pay up? The claim must be obvious, surely? Not always. This is why we have courts to decide issues that cannot be agreed between the parties. The claimant (the person making the claim) having to prove his or her case is the equivalent of the criminal rule that someone is innocent until proved guilty. In civil law, the defendant (the one against whom the claim is made) is not to be held negligent until either they or their insurers agree that they were, or they are found to be so by a court. Some cases are real battlegrounds and take several years to be argued and agreed or get to court. Some will be agreed early on and settled. Strangely, it is not always the very high value claims that are the most hotly contested. Insurers will often resist or try to reduce even small claims if they think the insured is not liable, or they believe that the evidence is not or will not be available to enable the claimant to prove his or her case, – or perhaps they think that the claimant will run out of money to pursue a case if they can drag it out long enough. However unfair it seems, that is the law as it stands.

Horses have a huge potential for accidents in almost any situation. It is impossible to make a definitive list of what will be a pure accident or what will constitute an incident which is someone's fault and for which in law they will be liable; each incident will be decided on its own facts. Even tiny and seemingly insignificant details can make the difference between something being no-one's fault or someone's fault, and following that the difference between a successful and unsuccessful claim.

If you do become involved in any sort of accident, first of all, if you are uninjured, make the situation as safe as possible. Get yourself and the horse off the road if it is a road accident. Do carry a mobile phone when riding, particularly if out alone, to summon help. Don't keep it on your horse's saddle – if the horse runs off in panic, the telephone goes too. Don't keep vital details about yourself or the horse – e.g. a warning of a particular medical condition – in your hat. Medical advice is not to try to remove a hat from a fallen and/or unconscious rider. If it is safe to do so, try to preserve as much evidence as possible. Write down what happened as soon after the incident as you can and date it. Get witnesses to do the same if they are willing and ask them to sign their statements. Identify everyone involved, including the horses. Can you describe the injuries, or if not, can you describe how someone appeared at the time – unhurt, upset, cut and bruised, seriously hurt? Take photos or videos, drawings or sketches of who and what was where – and where they ended up. Was everyone involved wearing protective or reflective clothing? Record the time, the weather conditions, the state of the ground. Get as much information as you can, because memories fade or alter very quickly. The

British Horse Society produce an accident report form which gives an idea of the type of information required.

Do inform your insurers as soon as possible of any incident that might lead to a claim. There will almost certainly be a time limit for this in your policy. If you wait too long before letting your insurers know, they may refuse to deal with either any claim you have yourself or any claim made against you. As long as you have informed your insurers in time of a potential claim, then it doesn't matter that a person making a claim against you does not decide to do so for many months. The insurers should still deal with it.

Your duty as a rider is to take as much care as possible to ensure your own safety and the safety of others, minimising risks and warning others as far as possible of potential risks. Of course, others have a similar duty to you: for example, drivers have a duty to respect you as another road user, and a show organiser has a duty to ensure that the fences that you are to jump are safe.

Legal concepts in accident claims

There are a few basic legal concepts that apply to all situations where an accident claim might be contemplated:

- Duty of care
- Breach of duty of care
- Negligence
- Causation
- Contributory negligence
- Limitation

These will now each be discussed in detail.

Duty of care

We all have various 'duties of care' towards certain categories or groups of people, even if we are not aware of it. Some are long established and will be well known: an employer has a duty of care to an employee, a driver to other road users, a doctor to his or her patients, a manufacturer of an article to those who might reasonably be expected to use it. Generally speaking, you have a duty of care to anyone whom you could reasonably foresee could be affected and/or damaged by your actions, either by you doing something you shouldn't, or failing to do something you should, if it was negligent for you to do or fail to do that particular thing.

The case of *Donoghue* v. *Stevenson* (1932) (All ER 1) set out the criteria that a court will consider when trying to decide whether a duty of care exists between one party and another. Apart from foreseeability, the court will look at whether the parties have a close enough 'relationship' such that one party would be in the other party's mind when considering whether their actions would affect them, and whether it would be fair to conclude that there was a duty of care between the parties.

As a horse rider and owner therefore, you would have a duty of care, for instance, to anyone riding your horse, to the spectators at a show, and to other horse riders where you are in a group or just hacking out with one other person. As a livery yard owner you have a duty to your liveries and as an instructor to your pupils. If there is no duty of care in the first place, then there can be no claim as you have no responsibility towards that person, or it may be that another person has no duty towards you. On the whole, if you can think of a way that your actions might detrimentally affect someone if you did something wrong, even if seemingly remote or far-fetched, then there may well be a duty of care.

For instance, say a farmer sells hay to a livery yard owner, who sells it to his liveries, and it turns out that the hay has ragwort in it. A horse dies as a result of eating the ragwort. The farmer may have a duty of care to the owner whose horse has died, even if there is no direct contract with that person. It is arguable that he can reasonably foresee that his hay was going to be eaten by horses and that if it had ragwort in it that a horse would be injured or even killed.

There are not many cases where it is argued that there was no duty of care, but this is possible. Usually it is accepted that there was a duty of care but it is argued that it has not been 'breached'. The duty of care towards a certain person or category of people can change according to the circumstances. In the case of *Ratcliffe* v. *(McConnell) Harper Adams College* (1999) (WLR 670), a student of the college suffered severe injury when diving into the college pool. The problem was that the pool was closed at the time – it was December – the student might have been drinking and he was not supposed to be anywhere near the pool at the time the incident occurred. The accident also happened late at night or in the early hours of the morning. The college argued that in those circumstances no duty of care existed from the college towards the students. Had the accident occurred during college hours, with the student being entitled to use the pool, then the situation might have been different and the college may well have had a duty of care. In this situation it was successfully argued that the student knew he shouldn't be anywhere near the pool, that he was not at that particular time under the care of the college, and that he was doing something outside his status as a student and therefore the college were not responsible for him at the time of the injury.

You also see this situation in employer/employee relationships. The employer is liable to the employee during the course of their employment and has a duty of care to the employee as long as they are doing the job they are employed to do. If an employee is off on what is termed 'a frolic of his or her own', then this is deemed to be outside the employment situation and there may be no duty of care by the employer. To put this in an equine context, suppose an employee is injured while riding the employer's horse. The horse is dangerous – it is a determined rearer – but the employer has not told the employee this. The horse rears and the employee is thrown and seriously injured. He or she may well be able to sue their employer (assuming negligence can be proved) as the injury would have been caused during an activity the employee was doing legitimately as part of their employment.

If on the other hand, the employee is injured while engaged in a fight over a personal matter with another employee, then the employer is unlikely to be liable for their injury. The employee has been injured outside the course of his normal and legitimate employment and an employer is not responsible for things that happen in that situation.

Breach of duty of care

If you can establish that there is a duty of care, which in most cases you will be able to do, before a claim can be made you will have to establish that the duty was 'breached'. In practical terms, this means that you will have to show that someone had done something that they shouldn't have done, or failed to do something that they should have done. However, it is not enough to show that there is a breach of duty. For there to be grounds for a successful claim, you also have to show that the breach occurred 'negligently' and that damage, loss and/or injury was caused as a result.

For instance, a motorist may well be in breach of duty towards you as a rider on the road by screaming past very close to you at 80 miles per hour. If your horse is completely unperturbed by this and nothing happens as a result, then there can be no civil claim as no damage or injury has happened as a result of the motorist's action, even though the duty of care may have been breached.

Negligence

The significance of the word 'negligence' is that if you establish that a duty of care exists and that the duty was breached, you have to go on to show that the breach was negligent. If it was a non-negligent breach then there can be no claim. When is someone negligent? Very broadly, they will be negligent when they do something unreasonable and can foresee that an accident or damage might occur as a result of that action.

Do you own a horse who you *know* kicks? If you tie it up outside a stable where you know people are going to be passing, and the horse does kick someone, then you are probably negligent. You know the horse kicks, you know there will be the opportunity for it to kick someone, and you can foresee harm if it does. Be warned – this may apply even if you warn people that your horse kicks. You do not escape liability by saying 'Well, I told you that might happen', and in fact it may have entirely the opposite effect. It is not enough to warn everyone else in your yard that your horse kicks and to expect them to keep out of the way. They probably will do so, however much resentment you cause by repeatedly tying up your horse in the way so no-one can get past without risking a good kicking. But supposing a child is around, or someone brings a friend to the yard who doesn't know your horse? It is your responsibility to act reasonably and not do as you like and expect everyone else to watch out for themselves.

As another example, you are organising a show and you note that the jumping arena has a number of large rabbit holes in it. You can foresee a horse putting its foot in a hole, falling and injuring itself or its rider, yet you do nothing about the holes. If a horse then does just that, you are likely to be negligent. It was unreasonable of you not to do something to fill in or remove the rabbit holes.

Are you riding in busy traffic on a horse you know to be completely unreliable in traffic? If it does panic, even when the drivers have done nothing untoward, and you are injured, it is likely to be your own fault – no-one appears to have been negligent but yourself. Similarly, if you cause damage to a car or a pedestrian as a result of your horse becoming out of control when you know it is likely to do so, then you may well be liable, notwithstanding the comment made earlier that the law recognises that horses cannot be controlled completely in all situations. The point here is that you are the one that has been foolhardy and negligent by acting unreasonably in insisting on taking a wholly untrustworthy horse out in traffic. It is not something that was unforeseen or that you did your best to guard against.

You may say, 'What about young horses, or reschooling horses or reintroducing horses to traffic when they have had an accident? Surely this can't mean that every horse ridden must be completely unmoved by all traffic?' No, it doesn't. The law says that you must take reasonable care at all times. Thus, if you have a young horse you should get it as traffic-proof as possible from an early age, either by walking it out or placing it in a field next to traffic, so that it is at least used to what might be termed normal traffic. When you first go out, have a safe older horse on the outside of you and pick quiet times and areas to ride out in until the horse builds up its confidence in traffic. Ride out at a steady pace and get off the road if you feel your horse is becoming a little unsafe.

Make sure you are visible. There is some controversy over whether you should wear a vest saying 'Caution – Young Horse'. Are you taking care to warn others that this is a horse that might do something unexpected, despite your best efforts, or are you implicitly saying 'I can't control this horse, so you'd better keep completely out of my way.' The key is still whether you are being negligent. You must not assume that by wearing such a vest you have licence to do whatever you want and everyone else must keep out of your way. If, however, you have taken every other precaution to ensure that you are riding your young or nervous horse as safely as possible, then the notice will probably be taken as one more prudent step on your part to do as much as you can to keep yourself and your horse safe.

It is impossible to say definitively when you will be negligent and when you will not. If you are faced with a claim against you or feel you have a claim, seek legal advice as soon as possible. The categories of negligence are not closed and probably never will be, as the law follows developments in real life. There have, for instance, been several cases where the Ministry of Defence has been found negligent for injury caused by low flying aircraft, and in the case of *Stiven* v. *Andrewartha* (1997) (*Horse Law* (1997) Vol. 2, Iss. 4) a low flying balloon was the cause of an injury to a horse and rider.

The plaintiff (who would now be called the claimant), a Miss Stiven, was riding a particular horse for the first time, though she had ridden before. A hot air balloon flew over her head and its burners were ignited, which caused the horse to panic. She was thrown off the horse and suffered serious injuries. There was some argument about whether or not she should have got off the horse to lead it, but British Horse Society guidance does say that the safest place to be is in the saddle on the horse.

Perhaps it is true that there is no definitive answer on this point and it depends on the circumstances. Sometimes it might be safest just to get off the horse and lead it away from the problem. There is some evidence to suggest that Miss Stiven did notice the balloon, but nevertheless carried on riding towards it. Be that as it may, she was successful in her action in as much as it was held that the balloonist should have kept a proper lookout before lighting the burners, and had not done so. Horses do seem to be quite perturbed about balloons, possibly because they can see them but can't hear them and find this to be very strange. You then get the sudden noise of the burners which may spook the horse.

One other point which came out of this case was the argument about whether the owner of the horse should have allowed her to ride this horse in the first place as it was prone to spook, but that line of argument was not followed. Miss Stiven was held in this case to be 10% liable for her own injuries by not getting off the horse.

Causation

A negligent breach of duty of care must cause some damage or injury for a claim to be considered. If no damage or injury results from an action, then there is nothing to claim for. Any damage or injury must be proved to have been 'caused' by any negligence.

Sometimes there will be a series of events leading to eventual injury or a worsening of an injury and in these cases you have to establish a 'chain of causation'. You have to show that despite some intervening event or events, it is still the original incident that started the chain and is responsible for the ultimate outcome. If an event 'breaks the chain of causation', then the extent of the blame to be put on the original person may stop at a certain point if someone else then becomes to blame. As an example, say you are at a horse show. The organisers have not checked the jumping arena and there is a large hole just in front of a jump. Your horse puts his foot into it and falls, throwing you onto the ground and breaking your ankle. It is likely that the organisers of the show will be liable to you for compensation for your injury as they have failed to take reasonable care to ensure that the arena is safe to jump in.

Supposing you then get taken to hospital by ambulance and on the way, the ambulance is involved in a serious road accident; it is not the ambulance driver's fault, but you now break your leg and both arms. There has therefore been an intervening event causing you further injury and this might arguably 'break the chain of causation'. You may therefore have two claims, one against the show organisers and one against the driver of the car that hit the ambulance. The show organisers may well be liable for your ankle injury, but it is arguable that it is not their fault that you were involved in an accident which caused you more serious injuries.

You could try suing the show organisers for all your injuries and argue that it was their fault that you were in the ambulance in the first place. If you hadn't been there you wouldn't have been further injured. The show organisers might then bring the car driver into the claim as a 'third party' to the claim, or alternatively, they might ask the driver or the insurers for a contribution to the claim to the extent that they were at fault. You cannot blame two sets of people for the whole of the injury and expect to claim compensation twice. Note that if it is impossible to decide which of two or more people is responsible for your injuries, then you may not be able to prove your claim at all because you cannot prove exactly who is at fault.

There is an interesting case, *Morris* v. *Solihull Health Care NHS Trust* (1999) (*Horse Law* (2000) Vol. 5, Iss. 1), which illustrates this to an extent. In

May 1994, Mrs Morris fell off her horse but was apparently making quite a good recovery in hospital. By August 1994, however, her mental condition had deteriorated causing her to be depressed and to talk of suicide. Eventually she did try and commit suicide by strangling herself and was clinically dead when found in hospital. She was resuscitated but had suffered severe brain damage and now requires continual nursing care. It is unlikely that she will recover. She claimed against the hospital saying that she had shown clear signs of suicide and the hospital had failed to monitor her sufficiently to prevent this. The hospital did not accept liability, but nevertheless settlement in the sum of £800,000 was achieved. It was not the fact that she had fallen from her horse that had injured her, so much as the hospital's intervening negligent act in failing to prevent her suicide.

It should be stressed that any intervening act must itself be negligent for any blame to attach. If it is not negligent, you can try blaming the originally negligent person for the whole of your claim.

Contributory negligence

Contributory negligence is a concept whereby you can be held liable to an extent for your own injuries by your own carelessness or neglect (Law Reform (Contributory Negligence) Act 1945). You can in fact be 100% liable for your own injuries, even where it is found someone else's negligent actions did cause the accident in which you were injured. Thus, if you are told not to ride a certain horse or told, for instance, not to ride it in a certain way, but you do so, then you are likely to be responsible for your own injuries. In the second example the owner might have liability for allowing you to ride the horse in the first place, but you may have negated this by not doing as you were told to do.

Supposing you were involved in a road accident and suffered a fractured skull because you were not wearing a riding hat. The accident might have been someone else's fault, but the injury you sustained might have been avoided, at least in part if not altogether, had you been wearing a hat. You are therefore at least partly to blame for your own injuries.

A car might frighten your horse but the reason you fall off is because your girth snaps due to your failure to maintain your tack in good condition and to check it before you left the yard. Had your girth not snapped, you would have stayed in the saddle. Again, you might be liable for at least part if not all of your own injuries. It is not necessarily the car frightening your horse that was the cause of your accident, but the snapping of your girth.

You have a duty to keep yourself as safe as possible and not take unnecessary and avoidable risks. Therefore, before you ride, check that your horse is sound and well and has no shoes loose etc., and check that your tack is well maintained, in good order and properly fitted, that your girth is tight and that all buckles are done up. Always wear a hat no matter how short your ride; do not even bring a horse in from a field without wearing a hat. It may not always protect you, and it will not protect you from a broken arm or ribs, but it may well be the difference between a headache or severe brain damage or death when a horse unexpectedly rears.

Wear a body protector and gloves and proper boots, to ensure that you have a proper grip on the reins and your foot does not slip through a stirrup if there is an accident.

Make sure you can be seen by others. Fluorescent riding gear may not make a fashion statement, but it ensures you are doing your best to make your presence known. It is surprising how easily horses and riders can blend into the background, even on a sunny day. Think of a dark bay horse in black tack, with you in a navy fleece and black jodhpurs, against a tall hawthorn hedge – invisible. Even riding a grey horse is no guarantee of visibility. Should there be an accident, if you are wearing bright and preferably reflective or fluorescent clothing and tack and proper riding wear, you will be given credit for having done your best to alert others to the fact that you were there, and to protect yourself from injury.

Limitation

There are time limits for making claims and you should stick to these. If you do not make your claim within the allotted time you will almost certainly lose your right to make a claim at all. Making a claim within a time limit means being in a position to issue and file all the correct documents in court ('issuing proceedings') if you have to, in order to protect your legal ability to make a claim within that time. It doesn't mean telephoning a solicitor to make an appointment to discuss your case. It takes a great deal of time for all the investigations and legal work to be done to look into your claim and issue proceedings if that is necessary, and it is no good going to a solicitor a week before your time is up expecting everything to be done at the last minute. You would be lucky to get a solicitor to take you on at all. If you are contemplating a claim, take advice as soon as possible.

It is in any case in your interest to make a claim, or at least to start investigations as to whether there is a likely claim, as early as possible while evidence is still fresh and events clear in your mind. Even if the advice is that you do not have a claim, at least you will then know this at an early stage and will not spend months or years wondering whether you should have done something.

If you are injured, you have three years from the date of your injury to make a claim. If for some reason you didn't or couldn't know you had suffered an injury at the time it happened, you have three years from the date you knew you had suffered an injury in which to make a claim. This is seen more often in clinical negligence claims against doctors or hospitals. Usually if you are involved in some sort of accident you will know that you have been injured, but there have been cases where, for instance, someone has had surgery and an instrument or swab has been left inside them. The person might suffer pain and/or perhaps infections for many years after but have no idea why, until perhaps they have to go in for further surgery or an x-ray is taken for a different reason, and the existence of the instrument or swab comes to light. They couldn't possibly have known before the real reason for the problems, so might then have three years from the date of finding out about it to make a claim.

If there is ever any doubt in your mind, or even if you have cause to wonder whether you have suffered an injury, go and see a solicitor as soon as possible and get advice.

There are cases where people decide to make a claim well outside the limitation period, even where they appear to have known or should have known of their injury. The court does have discretion under section 33 of the Limitation Act 1980 to allow a case to be brought even many years after the accident, where it considers it is fair to do so in all the circumstances. All the circumstances will include whether it is fair to the person you are considering making a claim against. There have been cases where potential claimants have been convinced they received an injury, but in the end discover the nature of the injury is different from what they thought; although they have suffered an injury and they know this, the real injury is totally different from the injury they thought they had suffered. The court might consider it fair to let them try and make a claim as they didn't know anything about their real injury.

As another example, you may perhaps have received wrong advice from a solicitor, who told you that you did not have a claim, but then many years later another solicitor tells you that in fact you do. Also, new evidence may come to light many years later that was not available at the time you could have made a claim, or in some extreme cases the defendants may deliberately be concealing some evidence from you that if known to you would enable you to make a claim. In all these situations the court might let you go ahead with your claim. It is not, however, safe to rely on section 33 of the Limitation Act and it should only be used as a last resort. The best approach has to be to take advice from a solicitor as soon as possible.

Note that the fact that a court allows you to bring a claim late does not mean that you have succeeded or will succeed in your eventual legal claim. All that has happened is that you have been allowed the chance to bring your claim rather than being disbarred completely due to the passage of time. You will still have to go through the legal process to prove your claim.

Children have three years from their 18th birthday to make a claim, i.e. until they are 21, as long as the accident happened when they were a child. If they are making a claim through the Motor Insurers Bureau, where they have been the victim of an uninsured, unknown or unidentified driver, then they have three years from the date of the accident. If they are under 18 they will need to bring their claim through a 'Litigation Friend' – someone who can in effect bring their claim for them. A Litigation Friend must always act in the child's best interests and is usually, but need not be, a parent. They do have certain responsibilities and a solicitor should explain the role clearly to you if you find yourself acting as a Litigation Friend.

If someone is very seriously injured and sustains a head injury or brain damage, or if they are elderly, perhaps with Alzheimer's Disease, or have another health reason why they are incapable of bringing a claim themselves, then the Mental Health Act 1983 comes into play. It sets out specific types of injury or mental states or conditions which in law render people 'incapable of managing their own affairs'. These people would need someone to bring a claim for them. It may be necessary to obtain a medical opinion as to whether the person concerned does fulfil the legal criteria for being incapable of managing their own affairs. Just being elderly would not necessarily be enough. The significance of meeting the criteria for this category is that if you do wish to make a claim, or a claim is contemplated on your behalf, then there may be no time limit on when you might make a claim. In law, it is said that 'time does not run'.

There are also certain categories of people said in law to 'be under a disability'. In this context, 'disability' does not mean a physical disability or necessarily a mental state making the person disabled. It is a legal term meaning that they are disabled from bringing their own actions under law. People incapable of managing their own affairs are under a legal disability. A child can therefore be said to be under a disability in law because they cannot legally bring a claim themselves. It does not always mean that the child is physically or mentally disabled, although it can do.

Say for instance, a child falls from a horse and is severely brain damaged, becoming incapable of looking after themselves and likely to remain so for the rest of their lives. If they did not have brain damage, then as a child they would normally have only three years from their 18th birthday to make a claim. Because of the brain damage, the child is both incapable of managing his or her own affairs and is under a disability. As mentioned above, 'time does not run' and a legal claim can be started at any time, perhaps even many years after the accident.

Physical disability alone does not render someone incapable of managing their own affairs, and the disability need not have arisen because of the accident for which the claim is being made. However, it is again in everybody's best interests for a claim to be made as soon as possible.

If you are the subject of a criminal offence, e.g. a drunk driver crashes into you or someone attacks you, you might be able to claim for compensation from the Criminal Injuries Compensation Authority. You have only two years from the injury in which to claim.

If you are complaining that you were injured because of a defective product under the Consumer Protection Act 1987, there is a time limit of 10 years and the discretion of the court does not apply.

Your horse cannot make a claim for its own injuries and neither can you make a claim on the horse's behalf for its injuries as such, because a horse is not a person in law. You can claim in a roundabout way for the horse's injuries in that you say that your horse's injuries have diminished or extinguished its value, and this is what you claim for. It is in effect a financial loss. You can claim for this up to six years after the event.

You also have six years in which to make breach of contract claims, i.e. sale and purchase claims. In some cases this can be extended, for instance, if evidence which would have enabled you to make your claim has been concealed from you deliberately by the defendants. This would be quite unusual, but is not unknown. You would need specialist legal advice if you thought this had happened.

Again, the golden rule must be to take advice as soon as possible if you think you have any sort of claim, not just an accident claim. Memories fade, evidence is lost, witnesses become unreliable, horses are sold on and it becomes more difficult to prove your case, which you must do if you are to be awarded compensation.

There are circumstances where it may be advisable not to settle a claim too early, e.g where you have serious injuries that will take years to resolve, but that is not the same as not starting a claim in good time. You can always begin your claim and use legal procedures to hold it up legitimately for a while where there is good reason to do so. For instance, you might be able to resolve the issue of who is to blame for the accident and whether the injuries you have were caused by that accident (liability and causation), but then agree or get an order from the court allowing more time to 'quantify' the claim – calculate how much your claim might be worth – so that you can see how your injuries are progressing. If they continue to worsen, then the amount of your claim might be increased. If they settle down or you make a full recovery, then your claim will stabilise.

You can get provisional awards, whereby you get part of your settlement but if you develop further injuries later you can go back to court for a further award. This can only be done where the court specifically says that the award is provisional and at the same time it will usually set out the types of injury that you would be able to claim for in the future if they develop. The further injuries normally have to be recognised complications of the original injury.

For example, say you have a severely shattered leg. It may take two and a half years to heal up but your surgeon is concerned that the circulation is compromised and the leg might end up having to be amputated. Your surgeon says that it could be five to ten years before they know whether this will have to be done. If your leg heals, you will be able to carry on with your showjumping career. If you have to have it amputated, it will change your life radically and perhaps result in a much bigger claim. Clearly you will not want to wait another five to ten years to settle your claim, but neither do you want to settle now if there is a likelihood of serious consequences in the future.

Assume that liability in this example is not a problem. The other side accepts that the accident was their fault, or your case has been to court and the court have found in your favour. You get an order from the court for compensation for the injuries you have suffered so far. There will be a clause in that order saying that it is a provisional award and that if your leg does have to be amputated within, say, ten years of the order, you can go back to court for future compensation for the extra injury.

Normally, once a claim is settled, it is settled. If you settle your claim completely on what is called a 'full and final settlement' basis, you will be very unlikely to be able to make any future claims arising out of the same accident or injuries. It is important to try to get it right at the start. There is a duty to put all available claims and evidence before the court at once. If this is not done, you may lose your right to make a further claim in the future if you missed out something that was apparent or foreseeable at the time and should have been claimed for.

From a defendant's point of view it can be seen that it is not safe to assume that just because three or six years have passed you are safe from a claim. Claims can arise many years later. While it is not suggested that you worry yourself about this on a daily basis 20 years after an accident, it can be worth gathering together evidence at the time that would enable you to defend yourself many years later. However, this can be a two-edged sword. If no evidence is available or it has been legitimately disposed of or destroyed (not deliberately with a view to avoiding a claim), then if a court is considering an application under section 33 of the Limitation Act to allow someone to bring a claim many years after the accident, the court may consider it unfair to let the claim be brought out of time if the defendant will not be able to provide a proper and fair defence due to a loss of evidence.

Procedure for claims

If you decide you may have a claim, get in touch with a specialist solicitor as soon as possible. The Law Society has various panels of approved specialist solicitors, particularly for personal injury or clinical negligence actions, and the Equine Lawyers Association maintains a list of solicitors and barristers with an interest and expertise in various aspects of equine law, not just accidents.

With personal injury and clinical negligence actions, the first step, once investigations have been carried out and there appears to be a case, is to follow something called the 'pre-action protocol'. This means that your solicitor will contact the potential defendant or their insurers in writing and set out your case in some detail. The other side then have a certain time in which to respond. They can 'accept liability', which means that they accept that they were responsible for an incident or injury, or that they are at fault in some other way; or they can 'deny liability' which means that they will not accept responsibility or admit that they are at fault. If this happens, you as the person making the claim will be required to prove your claim if you wish to pursue it, by gathering together supportive evidence and in the end persuading the other side or ultimately a court, that you do have a claim. The other side can accept partial liability, maintaining that you were at least partially responsible for what happened. In the case of injuries, they can accept that they did something wrong, but deny that their actions have caused you any injury or loss, or at least they can maintain that your injuries or losses are not as bad as you say.

The idea of following this protocol is that both sides get a good idea of what the other side is likely to say by way of claim or defence, and they give each other the opportunity to resolve a claim, or withdraw if there is no prospect of success, at an early stage before costs become too high. If, however, the matter cannot be resolved, then there may be no option but to 'issue proceedings' and begin a more formal claim in the courts.

The document that is issued, lodged in court and served on – i.e. sent to – the other side is called a claim form (see Appendix 6). The person making the claim is called the claimant. The claim form sets out the details of your claim in a document called a particulars of claim and may have supporting documents such as medical reports detailing injuries, other types of expert reports detailing why you have a claim, and a schedule of damages, which is a list of your actual and anticipated financial losses.

Once a claim form is issued, it must be served on the other side or their insurers or solicitors, together with any supporting documents, within four months of issue. If it is not served within this time, you may lose your right to go ahead with your claim.

Do check whether insurers or solicitors will 'accept service' – that is, are willing to have the documents formally served on them. They may not be and may want you to serve on the defendant instead. It is important to get this right. Service is usually done by post, using ordinary first class mail. Do not use recorded or registered post. If a person thinks they might be sued, they will be looking out for the court documents and could refuse to sign for them, thus avoiding being served. Be sure to leave yourself plenty of time to serve within the four months. Do not leave it until the last minute. You can serve someone personally, that is, by actually handing the documents to them, but this is not always satisfactory and can cause trouble. There are special rules as to where a company can be served – check on these at your local court. If you are legally represented, then of course your solicitor will be doing all this for you. If you are using the Small Claims Track, your local court staff will help you.

Once the claim form is served, the defendant has a certain amount of time to serve a 'defence'. This sets out why they think they are not liable. If they do not serve a defence within the time, then 'judgment can be entered'. This means that in effect you have won and can take steps to try to 'enforce judgment', i.e. by taking legal steps to get your money back or get compensation. Most people do put in a defence and in some cases, even if you apply successfully for judgment, the court can 'set it aside' if it is fair to do so.

Next, the court will set a timetable for the matter to get to court. Evidence will have to be exchanged before certain dates and a date fixed for a trial. Again, if you are represented, all this will mainly be your solicitor's job. A claim can be settled at any time before trial – or even at trial sometimes – but if it is not, it must go to trial and one side will win and the other will lose. Appeals are possible, but mainly only where the trial judge got things wrong either on the law or the facts. You can't appeal just on the ground that 'it's not fair'.

Chapter 15
Damages – What Can I Claim For?

The law can usually only offer a remedy by way of financial compensation. The remedy is available by successfully suing someone in a civil – non-criminal – court. Sometimes criminal proceedings can be instigated as well as a civil claim, but a criminal prosecution will not normally attract compensation for you, although the criminal courts do have power to make compensation orders. However, these will be unlikely to be anything like as much as you can expect from a successful civil claim.

A driver may be prosecuted in the criminal court for driving without due care and attention, or for dangerous driving, and may receive a fine and penalty points and sometimes imprisonment. This is strong evidence that an accident caused at the time was probably his or her fault. What the law can't do is specifically make, for instance, someone lose their job; the law is not meant for revenge. It is there to try, as far as possible by the provision of compensation, to put you in the position you would have been in if the accident had never happened. It can also try and put you in the position you would have been in had a contract been fulfilled.

Levels of compensation

It should be noted that damages for injuries are notoriously low in England and Wales, even where the injuries are extremely severe. There are no 'punitive damages' as in America where compensation can be set at a level meant to punish a person or a company for negligence; these are awarded in addition to normal compensatory damages for injury or loss.

The whole question of damages was considered in the Court of Appeal in February 2000 and it was hoped that the levels of compensation would rise significantly, but in the end they hardly moved up at all. Even for the most severe injuries – brain damage and severe paralysis – the top level of damages will be in the region of £150,000 to £175,000. It has to be remembered that this is the compensation for the injury alone. These are called PSLA damages, standing for damages for 'pain, suffering and loss of amenity'. The very high awards you sometimes see, amounting to millions of pounds, are made up of PSLA damages plus compensation for losses and expenses incurred from the time of the accident until settlement and for the future for a proportion of the person's life expectancy.

Every case is looked at on its own circumstances. Just because you appear to have a similar injury to someone else, you will not necessarily get a similar amount by way of compensation. It may depend on the effect that the injuries had on a person's life. For example, the loss of a finger for most of us would be disfiguring and inconvenient but we could probably adapt and cope. We would be compensated for loss of a finger and probably would be given something for loss of amenity, i.e. for the inconvenience in our daily life of losing a finger. The extent of the inconvenience depends on which finger it is. It would be more difficult to ride having lost an index finger than a little finger, for instance. However, to a professional musician or a brain surgeon the loss of a finger may mean the loss of a career as well. They may not be able to adapt at all to the loss of a finger due to the delicate and dextrous work they do. They would be compensated not only for the loss of a finger and the inconvenience, but also for the loss of future earnings that they could have hoped to have achieved. Thus their claim for the same injury would be far greater than ours because of the very different effect on their lives.

One of the most contentious forms of compensation is that under the Law (Miscellaneous) Reform Act 1947 and the Fatal Accidents Act 1976. It is sometimes said that it is cheaper in law to kill someone in an accident than to severely injure them; while cruel, that can be true. If someone is killed as a result of someone else's negligence, then by law the maximum award that can be given in respect of that person's death is £7,500. This is called the 'bereavement award' and is paid to certain categories of people because they have been bereaved of that person. It is paid to spouses of the dead person or to parents if it is a child under 16, or under 18 but unmarried. There is also an entitlement to the cost of funeral expenses for the deceased person. So if your child is killed in a road traffic accident while out riding her pony, you as the parent may only be awarded up to £7,500 for her death, plus the costs of funeral expenses. There is nothing payable under these Acts in respect of your own suffering, although it is possible that you may have a separate claim for psychiatric injury. To establish this you would need to take specific advice from a specialist solicitor. You may think that £7,500 is a derisory sum for a life; it is, but then what sort of money could replace a child?

If it is a parent who is killed, or a husband or wife, then there may be an additional claim for what is called 'dependency'. There are other categories of people who can claim under this rule but in all cases they will have to show 'dependency'. This means there can be compensation for the extent that certain people were dependent, financially or otherwise, on the deceased person when they were alive. As an example, say a mother of two children is killed. The widower will be entitled to a £7,500 bereavement award and the funeral expenses. If his wife had been working at the time of the accident, he may be able to claim for the loss of her income. The widower may have to give up his own job to care for the children, or he may pay for help to care for them instead. He may be able to claim for his own loss of wages or the cost of the help. The children can claim for loss of 'motherly services', i.e. the things that mothers do for children that cannot necessarily be fulfilled by paid nannies, however caring.

There is a case concerning the estate of a Mrs Lynne Stolliday (1998) (*Personal and Medical Injuries Law Letter* (1999) Jan.), who was unfortunately killed in a road traffic accident on holiday in 1995. Her daughter Katie claimed not only for 'loss of motherly services' but also for the loss of Mrs Stolliday's help to Katie in the care of her pony. It seems that Mrs Stolliday helped considerably with the work involved in keeping the pony. The judge accepted the argument that Katie would have continued keeping the pony and was likely to have replaced it with a horse as she got older. It was also accepted that Katie probably would have stopped riding on entry to university in October 2001 and the horse or pony was likely to have been sold. Mrs Stolliday's assistance with the pony up to that point was valued at £968 per year; the judge accepted that this would have continued for five years and so an award was made in the sum of £4,840 for loss of this assistance. Fatal Accidents Act claims can be quite difficult, so do seek specialist advice if, sadly, you are involved in such a situation.

Special damages

In respect of claims where someone is not killed but injured, we have seen that compensation can be awarded for the extent of the injuries, but you can also claim something called 'special damages' which relates basically to financial losses and expenses incurred because of the accident. Damages for the injury (PSLA damages) and for future losses are known together as 'general damages'.

If you are wondering what you can claim for under the category of special damages, a useful question to ask is whether you would have been put to a certain expense or suffered a certain loss if the accident hadn't happened. This is known as the 'but for . . .' test; you ask yourself 'but for the accident would I have lost this money/spent this money out?'. If a loss or expenditure can be related to your accident, then it may be recoverable. For instance:

- Have you had time off work because of injuries sustained in an accident, and not been paid during that time? You may be able to claim the lost earnings. If you get paid while you are off work, then obviously there is no loss, so you can't make a claim.
- Do you normally look after your horse yourself, but now have to pay someone to do it; or have you had to put the horse on full livery because you are injured? You may be able to claim the extra cost – the difference between what it normally costs you to keep your horse and what it is now costing you because of your inability to look after it owing to injury.
- Has your hat, body protector, saddle or other clothing or tack been broken or ruined in the accident? You may be able to claim the cost of a replacement.
- Has your horse been injured or killed? You may be able to claim the cost of your *uninsured* losses in respect of, say, vet's fees or the cost of a replacement horse if not covered by insurance. You could also claim any excess you have to pay on your insurance policy if you make a claim.

There are two points to consider here. Firstly, you have to look at 'mitigation'. This is the legal term for reducing your losses as much as possible. You are legally obliged to do this if you reasonably can. For instance, however hard it seems, sometimes it can be cheaper to put a horse down and buy another, than to continue having veterinary treatment for the horse. If this is the case then you may not be able to claim the cost of ongoing vet's fees from the defendant, the legal thinking being that you could have 'mitigated your loss' by having the horse put down. There is nothing to stop you keeping a very badly injured horse; the law does not say you *must* have the horse put down if cheaper to do so. It just says that if you do choose to keep it, you may not be entitled to look to the defendant for considerable and ongoing future costs for choosing do so. In reality, a court is usually sympathetic to a private individual who wishes to keep a much loved horse, and at least some of the future loss may be recovered. You may find a slightly harder attitude with regard to commercial concerns.

Secondly, in terms of a replacement horse, you may be restricted to claiming the value of your horse at the instant before its death. This may be less than the cost of a similar replacement or possibly less than you paid for the horse in the first place. You cannot better your position through your claim and hope to buy the dream horse you always wanted. There can be difficulties in valuing a horse that you bought for its 'potential', where it has not had a chance to display or achieve that potential.

Your horse may be severely injured such that his value is diminished but he still has some use. Therefore your claim will be restricted to this loss of value. It is difficult deciding on a horse's value. If the horse was bought for a specific long-term income-generating purpose, e.g. a race-horse or a brood mare, then you may be able to claim for the loss of the future income that the animal would have brought in. You may have been convinced that the two year old gelding you bought to win Burgh-ley would indeed have done so, thereby making your reputation as a producer of event horses and generating thousands of pounds, but it will be a lot harder to convince an insurer or a court of this. If you have a record of buying and producing young horses for eventing or showing, you will be more convincing than if this was the first youngster you had bought.

Even if you cannot convince the insurers entirely, you can sometimes be compensated for the loss of the *possibility* that it would have happened – the loss of the chance for the horse to prove itself. It helps if you have a full record of the horse's breeding, including any papers, and its history and achievements, plus photos and videos to show that the horse was indeed a good physical specimen with potential. Don't try to claim that a horse might have become something it clearly could never be.

If you are very seriously injured, you may be able to claim loss of earnings plus future loss of earnings, cost of alternative or adapted accommodation, cost of care, i.e. nursing help or general care to help you with day to day tasks such as washing and dressing, or special equipment – wheelchairs, remote control lighting systems, special beds, specially adapted transport. You can consider making a claim for almost anything that will help you cope with your disability.

If you do not bring in professional help your family can claim for the notional cost of the assistance that they give you. Note that they cannot do this if they were the cause of your injuries in the first place, e.g. your mother was the driver of the horsebox involved in the accident in which you were severely injured and the accident was your mother's fault. This is based on the case of *Hunt* v. *Severs* (1994) (2 AC 350). Another family member providing care would be able to claim. The family can claim the cost of looking after you at what is called the 'non-commercial rate', which will be a lower figure than the cost of you employing professional nurses and carers. Not everyone wants professional help and in some cases families prefer to look after people themselves. All these items can be claimed into the future.

There is an element of crystal ball gazing involved in this. Various experts try to predict how long into the future you will need specialist care or equipment or whatever, coupled with looking at your life expectancy. You cannot claim beyond your predicted life expectancy and you will not recover costs incurred for your entire projected life expectancy; the idea is that you are awarded a sum in compensation which, if invested at a certain rate, will provide income for you to meet your needs for your projected life expectancy.

Take loss of earnings, for instance. When the accident happened you might have been in a secure job with real promotion prospects, which you enjoyed and which you intended to stay in until you retired; or you might have been running your own successful business. The appropriate expert will try and plot how your career would have developed, or how your business would have flourished, given evidence from your employers or the history of your business. They will try and predict the income you would have achieved over a period and your claim will be for that amount. It is not an exact science and predictions can be difficult where you have, for instance, just started a new job, you are considering going into business or your business is very new. This is because there is little past evidence to go on.

Horse riders are known for being motivated to get back into the saddle as soon as possible, despite having some very serious injuries and disabilities. Horses can often act as great therapy. The cost of rehabilitation programmes can be claimed for and insurers these days are quite keen on rehabilitation if it means that a person can go back to work or in some way be less dependent in the future. So, in an equine context, consider claiming the cost of rehabilitation and perhaps training for a change of career. If you are in a wheelchair but have full use of your upper body and arms, could you retrain for a different career using your hands, say as a saddler for instance? Could you continue to run your livery yard or riding school by concentrating on the paperwork, employing a manager for the physical duties in the yard? You might be able to make a claim for this extra expense. Could you continue to ride and even compete or show if you had specially made tack, a totally reliable horse and a horsebox adapted for disabled use? Try making a claim for the cost of these. Do you need extra riding lessons to get back into the saddle because you have lost your nerve? Again, the cost may well be recoverable.

Don't think you have to give up if you are injured. It really is worth considering carefully how you can continue with horses if you really want to. You get one chance to make a claim; try and make that claim work for you and claim for anything that is realistic and feasible in order to try and put yourself in a similar position to that you would have been in if the accident hadn't happened.

You may be able to claim for loss of use of your horse as well, while you are unable to ride it. Again this is not an exact science and you may achieve say £20 to £50 a week as a notional sum to compensate you for being unable to ride your horse. If you have to hire a horse for some reason because your own horse cannot be used then you may be able to claim back the cost of this.

When it isn't worth suing

It must be stressed that it is only worth suing people who are insured or who have the means to meet any judgment for financial compensation. If the person you could sue has no money or assets or is not insured, they may not be worth suing. You should therefore establish as soon as possible whether it is going to be worthwhile suing someone. There is no point in suing for thousands of pounds a 19-year-old unemployed teenager with no assets or insurance. It is not worth suing him or her for £100; you simply will not get it, however much right is on your side.

It may also not be worth suing where the legal fees are likely to be higher than the compensation you can hope to gain. Although the general rule is that if you win your claim, your legal costs will be paid in addition to compensation by the losers, bear in mind that you are only entitled to 'reasonable and proportionate' costs. Small claims – those worth under £5000, or under £1000 if an injury to a person is involved – do not give rise to any costs entitlement at all. The courts now try to discourage people from spending huge amounts of money suing others for small amounts.

Recovering costs

In many cases the amount of costs recoverable is argued about and eventually agreed between the parties involved. However, sometimes both sides are so divided as to the amount of costs that should be offered or accepted that the matter of costs has to go back to the court to be decided. If this happens, then a formal bill will have to be drawn up for the court to consider, detailing all the legal work that has been done and the fees incurred that the winner is seeking to recover. The court has the power to 'disallow' the cost of what it considers to be excessive or unnecessary amounts of work, or to reduce fees if it considers these to be unreasonable or disproportionate for the type of case or the amount of money at stake.

The court will eventually rule on a figure that is to be paid to the winner by the losers. If, as the winner, your bill for costs has been reduced significantly by the court, you could find yourself in a situation where you have achieved modest compensation but the amount you are entitled to be paid by the other side towards legal costs has been reduced. Remember that it is you as an individual who is responsible for your solicitor's fees and you may be required by your solicitor to make up any shortfall when the other side have paid their share of your legal costs. Solicitors are not obliged to accept only what is paid by the other side; they can send you a bill for the whole cost of your legal action and expect to be paid. (This would not apply where your solicitor is acting on a Conditional Fee Agreement – a 'no-win, no-fee' agreement.). There is a right of challenge to your solicitor's bill, but the solicitor is the one to explain to you how to go about this.

Claiming from other organisations

Motor Insurers' Bureau

Motorists will of course usually be insured and if they are not, a claim might be possible through the Motor Insurers' Bureau (usually contacted via a solicitor). If the driver is uninsured or cannot be traced, i.e. found or identified (usually in hit and run accidents), the Motor Insurers' Bureau may compensate instead.

Criminal Injuries Compensation Authority

If you are injured as a result of a criminal act, you may be able to apply to the Criminal Injuries Compensation Authority (CICA) for compensation, particularly if there is no other way of achieving compensation from the person who committed the criminal act. The CICA exists to compensate those who are victims of:

(1)   Crimes of violence including arson or poisoning.
(2)   An offence of trespass on the railway.
(3)   The apprehension or attempted apprehension of an offender or a suspected offender, the prevention or attempted prevention of an offence or the giving of help to any constable who is engaged in such activity.

The above can include, for instance, someone setting a dog on you or attacking you. For example, if you are sitting quietly on your horse at a covert during a hunt and you are attacked by a saboteur or anyone else, you might want to apply to the CICA for compensation. Application to the CICA does have some conditions:

(1)   You have only two years to claim, even where the applicant is a child. There are some exceptions but these are rare.

(2) It is not necessary for there to be a conviction for the criminal act involved; the fact that the criminal act took place is enough, although the applicant must prove it did.

(3) You should report the act to the police as soon as possible even if you think there is no hope of finding or identifying the offender or of there being a conviction. You must also co-operate with reasonable police investigations. If you don't report the incident or co-operate, an award may be refused or reduced.

(4) If you in any way contributed to the offence, or have a criminal history yourself, the award may be refused or reduced.

(5) Applications are made on a form which you can get from the authority or from a friendly solicitor. You should submit as much evidence as possible.

(6) The Legal Services Commission Funding (formerly known as Legal Aid) is not available for these claims so you will have to fund any costs yourself. If a solicitor agrees to deal with the claim for you, they might agree to take their fees out of any award you are given, although beware of your legal fees exceeding any award. The authority might reimburse you for the cost of medical reports and for the cost of travelling to any medical examination at the CICA's request.

If successful you will be awarded a sum of money as set out by the CICA 'tariff', which is a list of injuries and what they are worth; for instance, a fractured rib is worth £1,000, two or more fractured ribs are worth £1,500; loss of a thumb is worth £15,000 whereas loss of an index finger is worth £7,500. Psychiatric injuries, scarring and burns are also covered.

In some cases the awards will be less than you might expect if you made a successful claim through the civil courts, but sometimes the CICA is the only remedy you will have in order to get anything at all. It is possible to make a CICA claim and a civil claim but any CICA award will be taken off any civil award, so it may not be worthwhile.

General points about compensation claims

- If you have an accident and you receive a payout from an insurance policy that you have taken out yourself for that purpose, say an accident policy, the amount you are awarded under the policy is disregarded when compensation is being considered.

- In other contexts, you cannot be compensated twice for the same thing. So if your insurance pays for the vet's fees, for instance, you cannot claim these from the insurer as well as from the potential defendant;

you can only claim for vet's fees above the amount your insurance will pay for.

- You may find that you can claim state benefits because of an accident. If you do so, then in some cases where you are awarded compensation these benefits will have to be paid back to the Department of Work and Pensions, and therefore the amount you receive in compensation may seem reduced. In fact the provision is there to prevent 'double recovery', e.g. where you are given Income Support to replace lost earnings to a certain extent and you also receive compensation for lost wages from the defendants. The amount to be repaid to the Department of Work and Pensions can be quite complicated to assess, but do ensure you discuss this with your solicitor. The Department will issue a certificate on request giving their calculation of the amount due to be repaid. It can be quite a shock if you have not realised that this repayment might happen and at the end of your claim you get far less than you were expecting.

- Be wary of being filmed without your knowledge. Many insurers now secretly video claimants to try to catch them out on their claims, particularly where injuries seem to be fairly slight but the claimant alleges serious disability and puts forward a large claim. It is not illegal to video you and it is usually done from a public place, even if you are filmed while on private property. However, there was a case where a person was filmed in her garden from the other side of the garden fence by someone on public land, but this was deemed too close and an intrusion. Surveillance agents are usually employed and they can sometimes sail a little close to the wind in the tactics they employ to try to catch you out. They have been known to let air out of tyres so that they can film you as the claimant bending down to inspect the flat tyre, or to follow claimants driving and turning their heads with ease, when the claimant has alleged that they cannot bend or turn their neck due to their injury. On the other hand, claimants have been filmed building house extensions when they claim they can do practically nothing and are wheelchair bound! Defendants have a duty to ensure that if they are going to have to pay compensation then it is in the correct amount, and that they do not overcompensate a claimant who is exaggerating the extent of their injuries. If you want to see a lawyer cry, suggest vaguely that you have 'good days and bad days...' in terms of how your injuries affect you. It is surprising the number of claimants who, when challenged, say they were filmed on a good day when you would hardly notice their injuries at all! Tape recorded evidence of conversations is not usually admissible as evidence where the person taped did not know they were being recorded.

- No one is going to punish you for trying to improve your health and your capabilities. A court will in fact be more impressed by someone making efforts to overcome their disabilities. If there is some treatment, rehabilitation or equipment that will help you, then ask your solicitor to try and obtain the cost of it from the other side in the case. An experienced personal injury lawyer may be able to make suggestions, but their advice will not replace medical advice and treatment. Ask your solicitor whether an 'interim payment', which is a sort of payment on account, can be obtained from the other side to help pay for this. If the treatment works then the cost will almost certainly be awarded in the end. If it doesn't work, then at least you will have tried. You may still recover the cost at the end of the day if it was reasonable for you to try certain treatments. Interim payments will be accounted for in any final award.

- Don't try and make yourself seem worse than you are in the hope of achieving higher compensation. You will almost certainly be found out, although it is true to say that some people do develop psychiatric conditions as a result of an accident, which seem to prevent them from improving or making a recovery. The law does recognise this problem as an injury, but it will need to be established and proved to exist with the assistance of psychiatric evidence.

Chapter 16
Paying the Cost of Legal Action

You may be wondering how you finance making a claim or indeed pay to defend a claim someone is making against you.

Private

You can pay privately if you can afford it. This means you pay your lawyer out of your own pocket for legal work done and expenses incurred. If you win, your costs, or the majority of them, will be recovered from the other side, but if you lose you will have to pay your own costs and the other side's as well. Therefore this could be an expensive and risky option.

Legal Services Commission Funding

Legal Services Commission Funding (formerly known as Legal Aid) is not now normally available for any claims that have a financial remedy, including personal injury claims or claims arising out of business relationships, contract or debt, etc. Such funding is not even available for claims for personal injury made by children. It is available for clinical negligence claims, but not veterinary negligence claims. This funding might in some cases be available, even where the claim is for damages, if it is in the 'wider public interest' for such a claim to be made, but you would need to discuss this possibility with a specialist solicitor.

Conditional Fee Agreement

If you wish to bring an accident or contract claim you will almost certainly be looking at funding it through a 'Conditional Fee Agreement' (CFA). You may know this as a 'no-win, no-fee' agreement – although this is not entirely true. You enter into this arrangement with your solicitor either at the beginning of your claim or at some point during the investigation of your claim. Under this type of agreement, if you lose you do not pay your solicitor any fees. You might still have to pay for expenses incurred along the way, e.g. medical reports and counsel's (barrister's) fees, but that will depend on the arrangement you have with your solicitor. You will also have to pay for an insurance policy which covers you against paying the other side's fees if you lose, as you will be legally liable for these. The payment for the insurance policy is called the 'premium' and is a one-off payment, unless you need to 'top it up', i.e. take out more financial cover if your case looks likely to cost more in legal fees than first thought.

If you win your case, your costs will be paid in the usual way by the other side, subject to them being 'reasonable and proportionate'. You may also get your insurance premium back, but there is much argument about this in the legal world at the moment and it may not be recovered.

If you win, your solicitor will take a proportion of any compensation you win on top of his or her basic fees, thus reducing the amount of damages available to you. This is called the 'success fee'. The size of this amount will depend on how difficult and risky your case is and how much risk the solicitor is taking on by dealing with it. The greater the risk and the more difficult your case, the higher the success fee. This fee can be recoverable from the other side if you win, but again there is some argument over this, and in some cases some or all of the fee may not be recovered.

It is extremely important that you discuss this type of arrangement carefully and in detail with your solicitor before entering into it. There are a number of different insurance policies on the market for this kind of arrangement and they will all have slightly different conditions. You should also be aware that the insurer does retain a degree of control over the case, because they have an involvement in that they will have to pay out if you lose. In many cases they will want to know that you have a very good claim before they will even allow you to take on the insurance. You can have a situation where a solicitor thinks you have a good claim, but the insurers feel it is too risky to go on or that it will cost too much when set against what you can hope to achieve by way of compensation. In this case the insurers can refuse to fund a case further and this might cause difficulties.

However, if you want to make a claim there is little option these days but to use a Conditional Fee Agreement, however unsatisfactory it may prove to be. In many cases these arrangements do work well. It is strongly recommended, however, that you go to a specialist personal injury/ equine lawyer if you are intending making a claim involving horses, whether an accident or otherwise.

Insurance

Do you have private insurance cover for legal expenses? You can buy a policy for this for which you may have to pay a fairly small sum each month. You may never use this insurance but if you do need it you will be very glad that you have it. Legal expenses cover might be provided within your ordinary household insurance so do check your policy and with your insurers.

Payment by other bodies

Do you belong to any club, trade union or professional body that will pay your legal costs? For instance, the British Horse Society provides for legal costs and the payment of compensation to others if you are a member and are sued in certain situations. Check your policy for exactly what the insurance covers – it may only cover accidents or claims arising in an equine context. The Countryside Alliance also, for instance, provide insurance cover. Be careful to check when your legal costs will be paid. Often, the legal expenses will only be covered where you are defending a claim brought against you, although there are policies which cover making claims. Check your own policy or ask your broker specifically about it when taking out insurance.

Chapter 17
Vets, Farriers, Dentists and Alternative Therapies

Horses have an endless capacity for getting themselves injured or becoming ill and as a horse owner you will become very familiar with the vet's car in your yard. There continues to be an increasing interest in alternative therapies such as homeopathic medicine, horse physiotherapists, horse aromatherapists, masseurs, black box practitioners and horse whisperers. We all know of the 'tooth man' and the 'back man' who appear at intervals and peer into our horse's mouths or push parts of their anatomy around. There is a certain mysticism to what they do. Vets and farriers have a long and complex training and certainly some of the alternative therapists will have a sound background – for instance, you cannot be a horse physiotherapist without being a human physiotherapist first – but others will have no formal training and will have no recognised qualifications or regulatory body to oversee them.

Sometimes this is because the particular therapy they offer is individual to themselves, or the therapies and treatments are relatively new and there are not sufficient practitioners or a long enough history of the treatment to be able to evaluate it objectively. They may be perfectly genuine or competent in their ideas and treatments; indeed there are many success stories, often at times when the more mainstream professions have given up and owners have turned to therapists as a last resort. Anything that improves our horse's welfare has to be welcomed. But how can you be sure that the practitioner you engage does indeed know what they are doing? What do you do when something goes wrong? How do you go about putting it right?

Vets

We are all familiar with vets, who undergo a lengthy training and are overseen by the Royal College of Veterinary Surgeons. All vets are either a member or a Fellow of the Royal College of Veterinary Surgeons. They are also governed by the Veterinary Surgeons Act 1966.

The Royal College maintains a register of veterinary surgeons and only those on the register, with a few exceptions, can practise as a vet and give veterinary treatment and perform surgery. 'Veterinary surgery' is described in the Veterinary Surgeons Act 1966 as the art and science of veterinary surgery and medicine, including:

• The diagnosis of diseases and injuries in animals
• Performing diagnostic tests
• Advising, on the basis of diagnoses
• Medical and surgical treatment of animals
• Performing surgical operations

Vets also have supplementary functions such as inspecting riding establishments and the regulation of animals used for scientific purposes. They have a general duty towards the welfare of animals.

Under the Act it is an offence to 'hold yourself out' as a vet, that is, pretend to be a vet or give the impression that you are in some way qualified as a vet either on a personal level, or in a business or commercial capacity. If you do this, it is a criminal offence punishable by a fine (Veterinary Surgeons Act 1966). You could not, for instance, call your livery stables 'Mrs Smith's Veterinary Stables' even if part of the livery business was given over to the recuperation of animals after illness or surgery.

To be entered on the Royal College's register, you have to qualify as a vet, usually by passing the necessary examinations. The register is in two parts, the register and the supplementary register. Those entered on the register are entitled to be registered as vets under the Veterinary Surgeons Act 1966. There are four categories:

• General List – those who have passed the appropriate examinations in the UK.
• Commonwealth List – holders of a Commonwealth qualification.
• Foreign list – holders of a foreign qualification.
• Temporary List – those qualified to practice on a temporary basis.

On the supplementary register are:

• Those qualified to practise prior to the 1966 Act coming into force.
• Those who have been on the register at some time in the past, but were not on it just before the Act came into force.
• Those who for seven out of the ten years before the Act came into force held a licence under the Veterinary Surgeons Act 1948, allowing them to treat animals for free, for example as an employee of a particular society or institution.

Only qualified and registered vets can perform such operations as docking (deliberate removal of bone from a tail) or nicking (severing of a tendon in a tail) and then only when it is necessary for the horse's health following injury to the tail. These operations are otherwise forbidden under the Docking and Nicking of Horses Act 1949. Only a vet can castrate horses, although castration of some other animals, such as lambs, can be done by someone other than a vet in certain circumstances. If an unqualified person carries out these operations it is a criminal offence punishable by a fine or up to three months imprisonment.

There are some exceptions whereby unqualified persons can carry out veterinary procedures or give treatment, but if you are considering treating your own animal other than for the usual minor injuries, it would probably be best to take veterinary advice at least. You should also check whether you would be covered by your insurance if something went wrong, or for remedial veterinary treatment if you are self-treating. Most, if not all, alternative practitioners should only diagnose and treat with veterinary approval and they could be breaking the law if they do otherwise. The problem with this approach is, of course, that many alternative treatments do not have much credibility in the veterinary world and many vets will not approve such treatments. This may be because of prejudice, but it may also be from a genuine belief that the treatment will not be of any use or may even be harmful. On the other hand, there are a growing number of vets who do see good results where accepted treatments have failed and who are becoming dually qualified – e.g. as a homeopathic vet or an equine physiotherapist. It may be something you have to decide for yourself.

Unqualified people can in some circumstances give treatment under the Act. The main exceptions covered are:

- Scientific procedures authorised by and carried out under the Animals (Scientific Procedures) Act 1986.
- Treatment given by an owner, a member of the owner's 'household' (what constitutes a household member is a question of fact and degree), or a person in the employment of the owner or a member of the their household. Thus, you or your groom could safely give treatment, but it is not suggested you contemplate major surgery.
- Treatment given by a person owning or looking after an agricultural animal as defined under the Agriculture Act 1947 if done otherwise than for reward, but with the exception of open surgery.
- Treatment given in emergencies for saving life or relieving pain.

If a vet administers a substance, there is an implication that the substance is safe to give. If it turns out that the substance is unsafe and it causes an injury or damage, then you may be able to make a legal claim against your vet. Your vet in turn might possibly have a claim against the manufacturers of the substance, as might you, but 'product liability' claims as they are known can be very expensive to pursue as they may rely a great deal on the provision of scientific evidence. The same implication of safety is not given in respect of alternative practitioners.

A vet will be liable for those in his or her employ. In the case of *Chute Farms Ltd* v. *Curtis (1961) (The Times* 10 October), a vet was liable where his assistant failed to give a yearling an anti-tetanus jab.

Disciplinary procedures

The Council of the Royal College of Veterinary Surgeons governs the conduct and discipline of vets and has disciplinary committees to look into disciplinary cases. Vets can be removed from the register of vets if:

- They are convicted of a criminal offence making them unfit to practise veterinary surgery.
- They are guilty of 'disgraceful conduct' such that it could be said to bring disgrace on the profession.
- They got themselves on the register fraudulently.

If a case is referred for assessment to a committee, there must be a 'legal assessor' of at least ten years qualification to advise on questions of law. A solicitor or barrister of ten years qualification would be suitable for this role. The advice of the assessor has to be given in the presence of every party and/or their representative at disciplinary hearings.

A vet can be legally represented at disciplinary hearings, which must be held, like court hearings, in public, the thinking being that justice must not only be done, it must be seen to be done. The public can, however, sometimes be excluded in the interests of justice. The disciplinary proceedings are like court hearings, with charges read out, witnesses heard, other evidence read, and judgment given on a majority basis.

If the charges are upheld, vets can be removed from the register, have their registration suspended for a time, or be given a warning. There is a right of appeal and a vet can apply to be restored to the register after at least ten months from the date of removal or suspension.

The fact that a vet has been disciplined by a committee does not mean that he or she is a bad vet and that you therefore have a claim for compensation. They might be disciplined for something completely unrelated to the way they practise. For instance, a vet could be removed for a criminal conviction for armed robbery. They could still be a wonderful vet. If, however, they were disciplined for continually being convicted for drink driving, and you could prove that the vet was a persistent drinker such that it impinged on his or her ability to perform his or her function as a vet, and that an injury had happened to your horse as a result of the vet being drunk and negligently carrying out surgery or whatever, then the disciplinary action might have a bearing. You would still have to prove negligence on the part of the vet, but a disciplinary sanction would be useful evidence.

Claiming for negligence

In the horse world, there are two main areas where we come across vets. One is in the pre-purchase vetting procedure, which is discussed in detail in Chapter 4, and the other is in treatment and surgery for our horses. In both areas, the vet has a duty of care towards you and if they are giving their services for payment, they will also have a contract with you. If you feel you have a claim, you will be seeking to show in law that the contract was 'breached' or broken in some way.

In any contract there are implied terms. This means that even if it is not expressly stated or written down, the contract will be taken to contain certain terms and conditions. Contracts can be verbal or written, but it is much harder to prove the terms of a verbal contract. One of these implied terms is that the vet will provide treatment using 'reasonable skill and care'. It is not possible to contract out of this implied term. If the vet falls below this standard of care then he or she may be negligent and thus in breach of the contract. If you can prove that the vet was negligent and in breach of contract, and as a result of the negligence breach you have suffered injury, loss or extra expense, then you may have the basis of a claim. Your solicitor should check whether you would be suing the vet personally or the veterinary practice.

Proving veterinary negligence is similar to proving negligence by human doctors. The same principles of negligence will apply to anybody treating or offering a service to your horse, be it a vet, a farrier or an alternative therapist. You will have to show that the person providing the service acted in such a way that no reasonably competent practitioner in the same field would have done, or failed to act as a reasonably competent practitioner in that field would have done. In human law, the 'Bolam Test' is used. This is the guideline by which the standard of care for doctors is judged. It comes from the case of *Bolam* v. *Friern Barnet Hospital Management Committee* (1957) (1 WLR 582). Vets and other practitioners are subject to the same principles, even though they work on horses and other animals. It would be a defence for a practitioner to show that even if all practitioners in the same field would not have acted in the particular way that he or she did, either in respect of an act or an omission, there is nonetheless a respectable body of opinion that would have acted in that way, even though that body is in a minority numerically. This is because the law does recognise that there are differences of opinion as to the way humans or horses should be treated, and there is not necessarily only one way to carry out a particular treatment. A vet or other practitioner will not be deemed negligent merely for making an error of judgement as to the horse's best treatment, where there are a number of treatments available, unless the type of treatment they chose was so unreasonable that no reasonable practitioner would have chosen that particular course of action.

The case of *Bolitho* v. *City and Hackney Health Authority* (1997) (3 WLR 1151) should also be taken into account. In human terms, this case says that if you are saying that someone should or should not have done something, then it is not enough to prove that it should indeed have been done or not done, you also have to show that whatever it was would normally have been done, as this was the only reasonable and logical course of action. A doctor or vet cannot, according to this case, escape liability by saying that they would not have followed a certain course of action where it would have been negligent to do so.

The case of *Calver* v. *Westwood Veterinary Group* (2000) (*Horse Law* (2001) Vol. 6, Iss. 1) illustrates this. Two veterinary experts were called, one for the claimant and one for the defendant, in respect of the standard of care given to a thoroughbred mare. The judge decided that he preferred the evidence of the claimant's expert and found for the claimant. The defendants appealed. They said that the opinions of both experts as to what should or should not have happened were equally plausible and equally acceptable courses of action, and so the claimant had not proved negligence. The Appeal Court agreed. So where you have two differing opinions on what should or should not have been done, both capable of standing up to scrutiny and being found reasonable, it seems unlikely that you will prove your case on the balance of probabilities, as you are required to do as a claimant. To succeed, it seems that one opinion will have to be illogical and/or unreasonable.

It has to be stressed that vets and other practitioners may only be subject to a claim where they are negligent. It is not enough to be rude or off-hand, careless or a bit slow. All these may form the basis of a legit-imate complaint, but they are not necessarily negligent.

The resolution of a complaint can be helped enormously by the keeping of good veterinary records. It is time consuming to make and maintain clear and detailed records, but it is time well spent. As a vet, if you can show a client, or solicitor, the exact instructions you were given by an owner, the examinations you carried out, the diagnosis reached and the treatment given, and all can be seen to be in order, then a complaint may either be resolved or just not pursued. If there are no detailed records, then the vet will not have any ammunition with which to defend him or herself and may have to accept a complaint where they feel they have done nothing wrong. There will be times when the vet record shows that something was done incorrectly or negligently. This can be looked at positively, as the least the vet will know at an early stage is that any defence is unlikely to succeed and perhaps an early compromise can be reached, saving costs and valuable time.

As a horse owner, you should also remember that desperate situations call for desperate remedies. A vet may have to make quick decisions in difficult circumstances based on very little information. Because with hindsight they were wrong does not mean necessarily that they were negligent. Remember that the vet cannot ask the horse where it hurts or what type of pain it is; they have to rely on what the owner says and their own observations, coupled with various investigative techniques where appropriate. Having said that, there are undoubtedly cases where vets and other practitioners do get it wrong and even if these actions do not go as far as formal litigation, they should certainly be brought to the attention of the vet's practice. Bringing shortcomings to light can help improve the service all round.

If you are seeking compensation it is not enough to show that your vet was negligent. You have to show that an injury and/or loss or expense has occurred due to the negligent act or omission, and that it would not otherwise have happened. Without this there is nothing to compensate for. In order to have a viable claim you need to prove that the vet was negligent *and* that this caused an injury, loss or expense. This is called 'proving causation'.

Proving negligence

How can you prove that your vet was negligent? You are not a qualified vet, so you cannot know what constitutes falling below reasonable standards of care. You therefore have to prove that the vet was negligent by obtaining independent expert opinion from another vet or similar practitioner in the same field. If the vet you are complaining about is a specialist in a particular area, say orthopaedics, then you will need another vet with the same expertise to provide a report.

The expert will be asked to provide an opinion on the standard of care reached by the practitioner complained of. In effect, the expert represents the whole body of available opinion as we cannot ask every single vet what they would have done in the circumstances. We use our independent expert as a representative of the profession. The expert's role is to provide an independent report and not to try and bias their evidence towards the person instructing them, even though that person will be paying the fee for their services. Their role is to 'assist the court with matters within their expertise', as stated in the legal rules known as the Civil Procedure Rules, which govern the procedures of legal actions up to and including trials. The expert should not think that it is their job to try to find a cause of action – a way to sue someone.

If there really is no case, either because the vet was not negligent and/ or because no injury was caused, then the expert should say so. Equally, if they think there is evidence to support a claim they must say so and explain why, and they must be prepared to support their view and give evidence in court if necessary. It is legitimate for an expert to change his or her view once they have seen the other side's evidence during the run-up to a trial.

The procedure for a trial involves the setting of a 'timetable' either by agreement of all parties with court approval, or by the Court itself, whereby each side discloses their evidence to the other side at a fixed date. Factual witness statements, expert reports, medical records and any other pieces of evidence you want to use are 'exchanged' with those of the other side. This is usually done simultaneously, so that both sides see the other's evidence at the same time, with neither side having the advantage of seeing the other's evidence first. The point is that both sides get to see and evaluate the nature and strength of the other's case. This applies to accident and other types of claims. These days, claimants and defendants are encouraged in a number of ways to be very open at an early stage about what their claim is and what evidence they have to support it. In accident and human clinical negligence claims, a specific 'protocol' has to be followed before you are even allowed to issue formal proceedings, the idea being that if you can see the strength of a case early on, you can make a judgement about whether it is likely to be successful or not. If there is no case, you will know at an early stage before too much expenditure on legal costs is incurred. If the case is strong, it might encourage early settlement.

If your expert does change his or her view on seeing the other side's evidence, this does not necessarily mean that they were wrong in the first place; it will often be that they can see the force of the opposing argument. These days, it is quite common for both sides to agree to use the same expert and agree to abide by his or her opinion. Even where both sides use different experts, the experts can be required, and even ordered, by the court to get together and see whether there are any points of agreement and where the real areas of dispute are. 'Single joint experts', as they are known, are more common in personal injury cases than in negligence claims, but are not unknown in the latter.

A supportive report on negligence and causation from an expert means that you will have the basis of a negligence claim; a negative report and your claim is effectively at an end.

As an example of negligence and causation, let us take the example of a mild case of colic in a brood mare. If the colic is detected early on, it will be entirely treatable and your brood mare will be none the worse. Say you find your mare at 9.30PM. Vets have a duty to offer a 24-hour service, either through their own practice, by a locum service or by sharing duties with other local vets. You ring the vet and he or she assures you that they will be with you in 20 minutes. An hour goes by and the vet does not appear. Two hours pass and still no vet. You ring the surgery and remind them and are told that the vet is on the way. Still another hour passes and no vet. By now your mare is seriously ill. Eventually the vet arrives some five hours after you first called them and by now your horse is beyond saving and has to be put down.

If you can show that the delay in attending to your horse made the difference between the horse being treatable and going beyond treatment *and* that the delay itself was unreasonable, then you might have a claim. The *delay* is the crucial factor. If the horse would have died or had to be put down anyway, say for instance because you discovered it in the late stages of colic, then despite the delay the outcome was no different. There is then no claim. You could still perhaps make a complaint to the surgery about the time taken to get to your horse, but in law you would be unlikely to succeed in a claim for negligence as the outcome would have been the same anyway.

If there is a viable claim, then what you can claim by way of compensation is basically the same as discussed in Chapter 15 on damages.

Human clinical negligence claims can be very costly to pursue, as can veterinary negligence claims. If you do have a claim, it is likely that the vet will be represented by the Veterinary Defence Union or an insurer. Vets are not obliged to have professional negligence insurance, so it is not always the case that any settlement you achieve will be paid by insurers. Most vets will, however, be members of the Veterinary Defence Union and as part of this, insurance cover is likely to be provided.

If a claim is made, the vet will inform the Veterinary Defence Union and they will look into the claim on the vet's behalf. Their advisory staff are usually vets themselves. They will not look into complaints made directly to them by the public. It is said that the Veterinary Defence Union will defend their members robustly no matter what. If this is true, then it is unfortunate that the attitude is so entrenched as there are undoubtedly cases where there is a legitimate complaint which justifies investigation and, if not compensation, then an explanation or apology.

The practical problem is that the Veterinary Defence Union can decline to settle claims early on and thus bring costs down. There is no incentive for them to do so. So you, as the claimant, have to pursue and prove your case as required by the legal principles of English law, running up legal costs and expert's fees and hoping that if you go to trial you will win and recover most if not all of your costs. For many the risk is too great and cases are dropped, wasting costs that have already been spent.

The Royal College of Veterinary Surgeons will look into complaints made to them, although they are mainly concerned with the professional conduct of vets and not, strictly speaking, negligence. They will make enquiries of the vet concerned and usually will pass on any correspondence from the vet to the complainant.

Sometimes the legal advice has to be that it is just not economic to pursue a veterinary negligence claim. This can be extremely frustrating where there does appear to be strong evidence of negligence. Many people say, 'Why should I have to prove my case? Why shouldn't the vet have to prove they gave my horse proper treatment? I've done nothing wrong, why should I have all the expense?' The basic answer is 'Because you do; it's the law'. It is based on the principle of individuals being innocent until proved guilty, although there is no concept of guilt or innocence in the civil law of negligence; those concepts belong in criminal law. A vet or other professional or practitioner is either negligent or not, based loosely on whether what they did or did not do was 'reasonable'.

Proving causation

'Causation' is proved on the 'balance of probabilities' test. This means that when we are looking at whether an injury or loss was caused by negligence, we are looking to see whether it was more likely than not to have been caused by it. Thus, if it could be said that there is a 51% or more chance of the injury or loss being caused by the negligence complained of, then your claim may well succeed – assuming you can prove negligence in the first place. If there is only a 50% or less chance, then your claim will be unlikely to succeed as it will not have passed the 'balance of probabilities' test.

The concept of 'beyond all reasonable doubt' again really belongs in the area of criminal law and means that there practically has to be certainty. It is perhaps more important to have a higher test in criminal law as if you lose in a civil claim you generally lose money but if you lose in a criminal case you are likely to lose your liberty.

Solving the problem without a claim

Although it is not suggested that genuine claims for negligence should be ignored in all circumstances, you may find that with a reputable practice which has a good client care attitude, you are able to resolve your complaint directly with the practice. This will depend on the nature of the person or practice you are dealing with. If you have a receptive vet who is willing to listen to your complaints and explain why someone that you think was negligent was not in fact so, or is willing to accept that there is a genuine complaint and perhaps offer an apology or something by way of compensation, then this approach will work. If, on the other hand, you are presented with a recalcitrant practice who refuse to believe that their vets could have done anything wrong, or that there is anything they should do by way of client care, then you are unlikely to get anywhere, or at least not without much expense and stress.

It is hoped that this comment will not encourage veterinary practices to adopt an unreasonable attitude in the hope of avoiding all claims. We all get things wrong from time to time; it is an occupational hazard. For this reason, as a horse owner it is probably best, if you can, to go to a specialist equine practice as they will have built up a reputation which they will be keen to preserve.

If you feel you have a legitimate complaint, try taking up the matter with the practice before you go and see a solicitor. Regrettably, although the writer is a solicitor, it has to be said that some solicitors will see only a potential case that will attract income, and may not have the necessary expertise and experience to suggest that a more informal approach might be beneficial.

In the first instance, you may want to write to the senior partner in a practice, marking your letter 'Private and Confidential' and setting out as factually as possible the basis of your complaint. It is often difficult to be objective as you can get quite emotional about what you feel is negligence towards your much loved horse, but pages of emotional vitriol will not at this stage be helpful.

Set out a chronology of events, what you think went wrong and what your precise complaint is. Send in any supporting evidence that you have, for instance photographs. You can state what you would accept as a remedy at this stage. You may want part of a bill to be waived, or merely an explanation as to what happened and perhaps an apology. But be aware that if you state what you would accept at this stage, it can be difficult to go back on that later and it can somewhat destroy your credibility unless you make it very clear that this is what you would accept *now* to resolve the issue, but you may not be so willing later on if the case is not resolved. Do not say therefore that you will accept something and then when the vet or the practice offers what you ask, think 'Oh, if they offer that, they'll probably offer more if I press'. They won't. It just causes resentment and can mean that what might have been a settleable dispute becomes a personal crusade on both sides and neither will give way. If treatment for your horse is ongoing, or there is an uncertain prognosis, it is probably best not to suggest a final settlement too early, but wait until the outcome is more certain.

Veterinary practices can help by explaining clearly to their clients in the first place what they think the problem is when they are called out, why they think that and what they propose to do about it and why. They should also give an estimate of cost where possible and practicable to do so (few people will be bothered about cost in an emergency – but this does not mean vets can charge what they like) and also the factors that may increase this estimate – extra tests needed, something unexpected found at surgery, etc. Vets could go as far as having written terms explaining what the proposed treatment is, what is involved, what it is likely to cost and factors affecting any change. If at all possible, the vet should telephone the client if the horse is being treated at the surgery and something unexpected happens or is found, to explain the problems that have arisen and may not have been apparent at first diagnosis and get authority to continue work. The client may want the option of ceasing work and putting the horse down on economic grounds. As the client, you can ask to be consulted in this way where practicable. Obviously it may not be possible in an emergency, and clients should not expect to be excessively consulted before the vet even looks at the horse. You do have to put your faith in your vet and if you can't do this then you need a different vet. Communication in laymen's terms by the vet is vital.

If the client and vet feel that they are both on the same side in wanting to help the horse, this will go a long way to avoiding complaints. If there is a dispute over costs, then it may be possible to have the bill looked at by an independent firm of loss adjusters to determine what would be a reasonable fee.

When considering a complaint against a vet, you may feel that you have developed a good relationship with your vet over the years and this is the first time that something has gone wrong, so you do not want to damage that relationship. Similarly, if the vet is the only one in the area, you would be in difficulties if that vet refused to treat your horse. It is not suggested that these practical considerations mean that you should be expected to put up with substandard treatment, but they are factors to be borne in mind.

Farriers

The Farriers (Registration) Act 1975 is the statute regulating farriers – those who shoe horses. Blacksmiths do not necessarily shoe horses; they can be just general iron workers.

The Worshipful Company of Farriers, under the Act, has the 'general function of securing adequate standards of competence and conduct among persons engaged in the shoeing of horses, hereinafter referred to as farriers'. There is a Farriers Registration Council which keeps a register of those qualified to shoe horses, and this is open for public inspection.

A person can only be a farrier if:

- On 1 January 1976 their name was registered on the register of farriers, i.e. they were a farrier on or before the date the Act took effect.
- They have been suitably trained or apprenticed and have passed a prescribed exam.
- They have trained as a farrier in the army and passed a prescribed exam.
- They are registered on part 2 or part 4 of the register and have passed a qualifying exam.

You can be registered in part 2 of the Act if, up to two years before application to go on the register, you have been a farrier in the army or regularly engaged in the shoeing of horses other than as an apprentice or during training. You can be registered in part 4 if you are not otherwise entitled to be registered under the Act but you have been regularly shoeing horses for two years prior to application to go on the register, or you have complied with apprenticeships and training regulations prescribed by the Council.

There is an appeal against refusal to register. Every person registered will receive a certificate for the part of the register they appear in.

The Farriers Registration Council have the power to approve institutes and courses for the training of farriers, and to supervise them. There is also an investigating committee and a disciplinary committee who decide whether someone should be removed from the register. Farriers will be removed from the register if:

- They are deemed guilty of serious professional misconduct.
- They were not qualified for registration at the time they were registered.
- They have been convicted of a cruelty to animals offence.

The committee can remove or suspend a farrier for a time. To have their names reinstated, farriers have to apply to the committee. Anyone not on the register is not entitled to call themselves a farrier or a shoeing smith, or to describe themselves in such a way that would make anyone believe that they were a registered farrier. If this happens it can be a criminal offence.

Only those registered can carry on trade as a farrier. Part 3 of the register allows people to be registered who only shoe their own horses or shoe horses other than by way of trade or reward. If you are registered under part 3 you cannot shoe horses 'by way of trade or reward'. This regulation does not apply to:

- Apprentice farriers (because otherwise they would never learn).
- People on approved training courses where farriery is involved but is not necessarily the whole training.
- Veterinary surgeons or practitioners.
- Veterinary students under proper supervision where farriery is part of the course.
- A person rendering first-aid to a horse.

Thus there is quite a high level of control in the farriery profession. Allegations of negligence are rare and it is very difficult to get a farrier to openly criticise another's work. There might be a slightly raised eyebrow, but generally if one farrier thinks another has done a bad job, he or she will just go about quietly correcting it. If you feel you have a genuine complaint about the standard of work of your farrier then you could contact the Farriers Registration Council, but as so often, possibly the best approach from a practical point of view is to take up the problem with your farrier direct, or just change farriers. The Council's website provides useful information on how to resolve disputes. Any formal claim against a farrier would be done in the same way as against a vet, with the need to prove negligence, causation and loss and the use of expert opinion.

Possibly much of the problem with farriery is that most of us do not know enough about it to be able to criticise. We tend to trust that our farriers know what they are doing (and usually they do) and it is difficult for us if we are not professionals to see when something has gone wrong.

There is an odd little case concerning a farrier. This is *R. v. Ronald Thompson* (1998) (*Horse Law* (1998) Vol. 3, Iss. 5) heard in Somerset and reported in the national press. Mr Thompson had shod a certain customer's horses for 18 years. He became ill and told his customer that he was cutting down his workload. His customer became concerned and turned to another farrier instead as she was afraid that Mr Thompson would not be able to cope. After changing to the new farrier, the customer started to find her horses losing an excessive amount of shoes, which she could never find in the field or elsewhere. She and a friend hid in the field over a week or so and eventually spotted Mr Thompson deliberately pulling off the shoes! He was charged with theft and convicted. He pleaded guilty and said that he had been worrying about his business, thinking that if the customer could be made to be dissatisfied with the new farrier, she would return to him – quite a sad case really.

Dentists

There are no equine 'dentists' as such at the time of writing. Until 2001 in the UK, there was no qualification in equine dentistry and no specific training courses. There were in America but American qualifications are not recognised in Britain. We have the British Veterinary Dentists Association and also the Worldwide Association of Equine Dentistry (UK). The British Equine Veterinary Association (BEVA) have now set up proper dentistry examinations and the first group of practitioners have passed the examination leading to a qualification as an equine dental technician. They can also become members of the British Association of Equine Dental Technicians. Therefore, the correct term is not 'horse dentist' and anyone who says they are a qualified horse 'dentist' may not be. The dentistry examination covers examining the horse, assessment for treatment and actual treatment, dental charting, dental anatomy and pathology, use of instruments, hygiene, infection, safety, horse handling and written and oral advice to clients.

Vets are qualified to work on horses' teeth. A person who is not a vet or a qualified technician is limited to being able to rasp teeth. The traditional tools for horse dentistry are a gag to hold the mouth open, a selection of files and rasps and a bucket of water to dip them in between horses. We are now seeing the growth of the use of electric tools, such as rasps, which are clearly quicker and more efficient but are also likely to cause more damage in the wrong hands. Hopefully, the new examination and qualification will mean that only qualified people will use these now. If a horse needs extensive dentistry work where it would be more efficient to use an electric rasp, he will need to be sedated. Only vets can inject horses or give sedation, so if your horse needs this type of work, you will either have to take the horse to the vet's premises where the dentist may be holding a clinic, or the vet and the dentist will have to come to you so that the vet can sedate your horse at home and possibly wait while the dentist does the necessary work in case there are any problems.

There is little doubt that horse dentistry will be a growth area, and a good thing too if it leads to more comfortable horses. At the moment, however, if something goes wrong, as with vets, you have to take it up under the ordinary principles of law of negligence and causation and/or contract with the practitioner themselves, as usually they are individuals on a self-employed basis. In the usual way, they have a contract with you and just like any other person offering a service, there is an implied term that the work will be carried out with reasonable care and skill. If that term is breached and damage occurs, there may be a possible claim in the same way as there would be against a vet. If the person is employed by someone else, for instance a veterinary surgery, then the employer may be liable for their actions and your complaint should be directed there. You should also now be able to complain to the new British Association of Equine Dental Technicians if the practitioner is a member.

You should check that the equine dental technician is insured against claims, although almost certainly they will be. The problem, as with vets, should you be considering a claim, is one of economics. Unless the damage done is extensive, severely affecting the performance of your horse and therefore the value of him, or the damage requires prolonged and extensive remedial treatment to put right, any claim is likely to be well under the Small Claims Track limit of £5,000 and possibly uneconomic to pursue. Because there are so few practitioners you may also find it difficult to find expert opinion as to whether the dentist has been negligent or not. Hopefully, however, formal litigation will not be necessary.

Alternative practitioners

Herbalists, horse physiotherapists, Shiatsu practitioners, equine clairvoyants and other alternative practitioners can all have something to offer and generally show some evidence of success, but the comments on equine dental technicians in the last section also apply here. How do you get a remedy when something goes wrong and how do we measure the quality of their treatment when there may be few if any similar practitioners?

Alternative therapists are subject to the same principles that have gone before, i.e. reasonable care and skill, but it is suggested in these situations that the watchword should be caution before you allow someone to work on your horse. Do remember that they should only work under the supervision of a vet and with your vet's knowledge and consent. This does not mean that the vet has to be physically in the yard when the treatment is being given, but the vet should know of the proposed treatment and the outcome. In many cases, the therapist will only work after consulting with your vet. There may be something in your horse's health history that they need to be aware of and which would affect their treatment. If the therapist does not ask for the vet's consent, then do mention it to them, particularly if your horse is still being treated by the vet or is on medication.

Consult with your vet before trying new therapies, but be aware that many vets will have a healthy cynicism about alternative treatments, largely because in many cases there will be no hard scientific evidence of their usefulness. Having said that, many insurers do now pay out for alternative treatments, so they are gaining in credibility. Check whether your insurance covers you before embarking on the treatment, if you want to claim the cost back. A vet's recommendation might be required.

If the treatment offered by the alternative therapist is non-invasive and unlikely to do any harm, even if it doesn't do any good, then it may be worth trying. Sometimes treatments do work but no-one can explain why. However, where the treatment is likely to be quite invasive and could cause damage if it went wrong, you should think carefully before embarking on it. Don't forget that there is not the same implication that substances administered will be safe, as there is with vets.

It may be that you have turned to alternative therapists as a last desperate remedy, in which case you have little to lose, but it is always worth asking whether you can talk to other clients of the practitioner to see if they have been satisfied. A genuine practitioner will be only too keen to let you talk to other satisfied customers and if there is some reluctance then you should tread carefully.

A diligent therapist will take a full history of the horse – any falls, injuries, illnesses, medication, ridden problems, diet, etc. They may want to see the horse's tack and even see the horse ridden or lunged if possible. It is helpful if there is a hard surface to test the horse, on as well as a school. The therapist should explain what they are doing and why and should give clear follow-up instructions. Vets should do all this as well.

Always check that your alternative practitioner is insured against anything going wrong. It is the writer's experience, both in human and equine negligence claims, that alternative therapists feature very little, but whether this is because they are extremely expert or because sufficient treatment is not done for there to be a significant number of complaints, is open to argument.

Courses in new ideas

Hand in hand with new ideas in treatment and therapy are courses to teach you about them and to teach you new methods of horsemanship. This is all to the good in theory. There is no one way of dealing with horses, and different methods will suit different people and horses. But you would be advised to approach these courses with an open mind and perhaps not expect too much from them, particularly shorter courses designed as introductions to new ways of thinking. The people running these courses will usually have many years experience with all types of horses and handling methods and will have achieved their level of expertise over many years of commitment. Therefore, do not expect to be able to complain and get your money back if you return full of enthusiasm about handling your horse after a weekend learning the basics, and your horse has other ideas. These methods often require much time and specific equipment and will not work successfully without the right conditions. This is not the fault of those advocating new ways of thinking; it is just how it works.

If you are advertising such a course, in order to avoid complaints be very clear what the course is for and what can be expected, both in any literature and in any introduction to the course. Generally speaking, the longer the course and the more it costs, the more attenders will expect to achieve. The wording of advertisements is usually seen in legal terms as a 'mere puff' – encouraging wording designed to attract custom but perhaps not entirely accurate. However, it can become part of the terms and conditions of a contract, as can the wording of any brochures or literature, so be careful of the claims made. Clients will always be happier to have expected less and received more than the other way round, and happy clients are your best advertisement.

Chapter 18
Animal Welfare

According to the European Union, animals have the right to five freedoms:

- The freedom from hunger and thirst
- The freedom to be protected from the environment
- The freedom from fear and distress
- The freedom from disease and pain
- The freedom to exhibit normal behaviour patterns.

No-one could argue against these principles as a basic minimum for the welfare of animals. Most horses are cared for by devoted owners to a standard many humans can only dream of. If there is a warmer rug, a more digestible feed, a comfier saddle, a kinder bit – horse owners have to have it. Our horses' teeth are filed, their backs manipulated, their shoes hand-made and replaced regularly, their diet balanced, etc.

Who could be cruel to a horse? They trust us to provide for them – they have to, as we put them into an artificial environment where they are not able to fend for themselves; they often do not have access to constant grazing or running water, and they do not live in a herd; we ask them to go in trailers and to jump and perform dressage movements at our request. On the other hand, we free them from having to face harsh winters on a moor, from yearly pregnancies, from injuries incurred from fighting to maintain their place in the herd. For the most part it works. Humans and horses lead a happy co-existence.

Cruelty and negligence do exist, but often are due to ignorance rather than intent. We have learnt a lot – for instance, the Monty Roberts method of leading a horse into work gently, making him want to please you. Many people now refer to 'breaking' as 'starting', to reflect the kinder attitude to initial training these days. There is a vociferous animals rights movement, maintaining that animals have the same rights as humans. There is a body of opinion that seeks to have fox hunting banned.

One of the problems with cruelty cases is in deciding what does and does not constitute cruelty. For instance, it might be just as cruel and thoughtless to overfeed a horse as underfeed it, but generally, the Royal Society for the Prevention of Cruelty to Animals (RSPCA) does not receive phone calls complaining of horses being too fat. They do receive complaints of underfed and thin horses, and sometimes these are horses that are not being ill-treated at all – they are just extremely fit and lean. Cruelty can be very subjective. Different people and organisations will hold different opinions as to what is acceptable in horse care. Is it better to leave a horse out, even in the worst weather, because it is more 'natural' or should we bring them in in November and not let them see light of day again until the spring grass is through? Different people have different ideas.

The law does offer animals some protection – or allows heavy-handed interference some people would say – but there is plenty of room for education rather than prosecution.

Laws protecting animals

The main law relied on is the Protection of Animals Act 1911, but there are others. The Docking and Nicking of Horses Act 1949 is an Act to 'restrict the docking and nicking of horses and the importation of docked horses'. This practice is now prohibited except for health reasons. Horses are rarely, if ever, used in scientific experiments, but if they were the Animals (Scientific Procedures) Act 1986 would apply. The Act sets out protective criteria for animals that are so used. The Riding Establishments Acts 1964 and 1970 set out standards to be reached before riding schools can be licensed, and the Farriers (Registration) Act 1975 regulates those who can shoe horses. The Abandonment of Animals Act 1960 makes it an offence to abandon an animal temporarily 'in circumstances likely to cause the animal any unnecessary suffering'. The Cruel Tethering Act 1988 strives to prevent cruel tethering.

Protection of Animals Act

Under the Protection of Animals Act 1911 the offences that are mainly relevant to horses are set out in section 1. Section 1(i) says:

- 'if any person shall cruelly beat, kick, ill treat, over-ride, over-drive, over-load, torture, infuriate, or terrify any animal, or shall cause or procure, or, being the owner, permit any animal to be so used, or shall, by wantonly or unreasonably doing or omitting to do any act, or causing or procuring the commission or omission of any act, cause any unnecessary suffering, or being the owner, permit any unnecessary suffering to be so caused to any animal, or:

- shall convey or carry, or cause or procure, or, being the owner, permit to be conveyed or carried, any animal in such manner or position as to cause that animal any unnecessary suffering, or:
- shall wilfully, without any reasonable cause or excuse, administer, or cause or procure, or being the owner, permit, such administration of, any poisonous or injurious drug or substance to any animal, or shall wilfully, without any reasonable cause or excuse, cause any such substance to be taken by any animal, or:
- shall subject, or cause or procure, or being the owner permit, to be subjected, any animal to any operation which is performed without due care and humanity, or:
- shall tether any horse, ass or mule under such conditions or in such manner as to cause that animal unnecessary suffering,

such person shall be guilty of an offence of cruelty within the meaning of this Act.'

If you are convicted of an offence under this Act, the case will usually be heard in the magistrates' court and you can be liable to imprisonment for up to six months or a fine. An owner shall be deemed to have permitted cruelty within the meaning of the Act if he has failed to exercise 'reasonable care and supervision in respect of the protection of the animal', but where you have been convicted of having *permitted* cruelty rather than actually inflicting it yourself, then before you can be imprisoned you must be given the option of paying the fine.

The Act creates a large number of possible offences and each one can be a separate offence. You do not therefore have to be found guilty of cruelly beating *and* kicking *and* ill-treating a horse to be convicted; just one of the actions can give rise to a prosecution. If the accusations are all the same but relate to several horses, there may only be one conviction rather than a conviction for each horse.

The majority of criminal offences require the act creating the offence to be performed *and* the offender to intend that it should be. But with the exception of the offence of administering harmful substances, the Protection of Animals Act does not necessarily require any cruelty to be intentional for a possible offence to be committed and in some cases intent will not need to be proved. However, for the offences of 'causing or procuring', the cruelty, mental intent, or 'guilty knowledge' must be shown. Having said that, if there is 'factual' cruelty, or cruelty so obvious that no-one could mistake it for anything else, the intention may become irrelevant.

There can be difficulties in proving that someone did know that they were causing unnecessary suffering, particularly where they are accused of failing to do something and as a result a horse suffers. They may not have appreciated the nature or severity of a situation. Many horses will 'switch off' if they are in pain and give the impression of just being quiet. Livery yard owners should be aware of the possibility of an offence being committed where they knowingly allow an owner to ill-treat or neglect a horse and fail to do anything about it.

'Unnecessary suffering' has been referred to as 'suffering that is not inevitable in that it can be terminated or alleviated by an objective reasonably practicable measure'. Thus, objectively, it would be both reasonable and practicable for a farrier to be called to treat a horse with over-long hooves and it may be no defence to say that you could not afford to. That is a subjective reason, a reason personal to you. It may be an explanation, but it may not be a defence. The key is the 'unnecessary' element of the suffering. Regrettably (though fortunately, these are becoming fewer and less acceptable) there are situations where suffering will be inflicted but will be considered justifiable – horses in war, for instance.

At the moment the Act does not protect animals who are subject to research under the Animals (Scientific Procedures) Act 1986, nor does it apply to any actions in the course of destruction or preparation for destruction of an animal as food for humans unless such destruction or preparation was 'accompanied by the infliction of unnecessary suffering'.

Under section 2 of the Protection of Animals Act, where an owner is convicted of cruelty, the court can order that the horse be destroyed if it would be cruel to keep it alive. Before the court can do this, it needs evidence from a vet. It can also order the costs of destruction to be paid by the owner.

Under section 3 the court can, if it thinks that the horse would be exposed to further cruelty if left with the owner, 'deprive such person of the ownership of the animal and may make such order as to the disposal of the animal as they think fit under the circumstances'. The court cannot make such an order unless it has evidence that the owner has previous similar convictions or has evidence 'as to the character of the owner' or 'otherwise'. These phrases give rise to the possibility of all sorts of interpretations and allow the court to consider almost any evidence it chooses.

Under the Protection of Animals (Amendments) Act 1954, the court has the power to disqualify anyone convicted of cruelty from keeping a horse (if their offence and conviction is of cruelty to a horse; they could disqualify them from keeping a dog if the offence was against a dog, etc.) for 'such period as they think fit' in addition to any other punishment. This order can be suspended for a time to enable arrangements to be made for the horse to be looked after for the period of disqualification.

If a person is so disqualified, then after 12 months from the date of the order, he or she can apply to have the disqualification removed. When deciding if a ban on keeping horses (or indeed other animals if the conviction was for other animals) should be lifted, the court will, if it considers it proper to do so, consider the character of the applicant or the conduct of that person since the order was imposed. They will also look at the nature of the original offence and 'any other circumstances of the case'. If you breach a ban made by the court, then this in itself is a further offence with imprisonment and/or a fine as a punishment. Welfare societies often have to bear the cost of keeping animals where the owner is banned from keeping animals but refuses to let the society take over ownership of the animal. They may have no option but to return the animal at the end of the ban.

Section 5 of the Act allows a 'constable' to enter a knacker's yard 'at any time in the day or when business is being carried on' to see whether there is any contravention of the Act. For the purposes of the Act, the knacker becomes the 'owner' of the horses sent to him.

Section 11 states that if a police constable finds any animal so diseased, so severely injured, or in such a physical condition that, having regard to the means available for removing the animal, there is in the constable's opinion no possibility of removing it without cruelty, then he or she can authorise the destruction of the horse on veterinary advice that it would be cruel to keep it alive. This can only be done in the absence of the owner or where the owner refuses to consent to the destruction when a vet has been called and has so certified. In this situation, destruction can be undertaken without the consent of the owner.

If it is possible to move the horse without cruelty, again on veterinary advice, then this must be done by 'the person in charge of the animal' as soon as possible. This may not be the same person as the owner. If the horse is not moved, then the constable can do so without consent. Any expenses incurred in destruction or removal can be recovered from the owner as a normal debt, through the civil courts if necessary.

Section 12 allows a police constable to 'apprehend without warrant' a person who he has reason to believe is guilty of an offence under the Act, which is 'punishable by imprisonment without the option of a fine' – i.e. usually not an offence under section 2 whereby an owner has permitted cruelty by failing to exercise care and supervision. The police constable needs to have cause to believe that an offence is being committed, either as a result of forming this view him or herself, or upon a complaint being made about the horse.

The constable can also under this section take charge of the horse and 'deposit the same in some place of safe custody' – usually with an animal welfare society – pending investigations and/or ultimately proceedings.

It can be seen that there is scope for personal opinion in forming views as to whether or not an offence is being committed and it may be possible to challenge those views as the basis of a defence, or the opposite, if you do get caught up in a prosecution.

The law can be frustrating, as it does not allow you as a member of the public to legally 'rescue' a horse or pony, even where you can see that there is apparent suffering. You might, for instance, know of a horse apparently abandoned in a field with no grazing and no fresh water provided. You cannot take the horse into your own care – this could be theft. If you take over care of the horse in your own time and at your own expense, then you are helping a possibly uncaring owner to carry on keeping horses in a completely inadequate way and you are thus actually making the long-term situation worse.

Welfare organisations

The RSPCA and bodies such as the International League for the Protection of Horses can provide any number of heart-breaking stories of horses up to their knees in their own filth, foals standing starving over dead mothers, and horses, ponies and donkeys unable to stand because of overgrown hooves, and in many cases there is little they can do by way of legal enforcement because they have to wait until the suffering is so bad that a conviction for cruelty is likely. There is no easy answer and meanwhile horses continue to suffer. However, if you do get involved certain procedures must be adhered to in order to ensure that you do not find yourself on the receiving end of a prosecution. You would think that those who ill-treat horses would be too ashamed to attack those who have tried to help their horse. But they are often the ones most concerned to assert their 'rights', even where those rights seem to include the right to keep horses in misery.

In the case of RSPCA v. *Probert* (1996) (*Horse Law* (1998) Vol. 2, Iss. 2, *The Times*, (1997) 1 February), the defendant was convicted of cruelty to a Welsh cob and fined. The cob had been placed with a welfare society pending prosecution, but on conviction no order was made against the defendant that the cob should be forfeited. Mr Probert wanted his cob back. The welfare society refused to give it back and Mr Probert sued for its return. The welfare society were wrong not to give the cob back and the court found in favour of Mr Probert in principle. They did not let him have the cob back, however. The welfare society were ordered to pay him damages of £250 and were allowed to keep the cob.

This is not to say that the defendant in this case *would* have continued causing suffering to the horse had he been returned. His conviction may have been the result of a one-off unfortunate incident and he was now quite capable of looking after the horse. If that were the case, then it is only right that he should have the opportunity of getting his horse back. Clearly, however, the court were unhappy to return the horse to him. From either point of view there are risks in this approach. In such a case, if the defendant sued they might not get their horse back and they might incur legal costs, ending up with only a small amount of damages. The welfare society would have to consider the risks of illegally keeping the horse in the hope that the rightful owner would not sue, and if the owner did sue, the risk that they would have to pay large legal costs and compensation, while seeing the horse go back to what they considered an unsuitable home.

The different welfare bodies hold different views of how the problem should be tackled. Not all suffering is as a result of deliberate cruelty; much arises out of ignorance and lack of education. The International League for the Protection of Horses, for instance, tend towards an ethos of raising awareness of cruelty, education and rehabilitation, whereas the RSPCA are more inclined to try to prevent cruelty by prosecutions. There is room for both approaches and the welfare societies do work together in some cases.

Investigation by RSPCA

None of the staff of any of the welfare bodies have any more authority to arrest people, enter private land, search properties or seize animals than any other member of the public, which is to say they have practically none. The RSPCA does have a 'protocol' – procedural guidelines – for investigations and recording of equine welfare issues. They do not have any right to enter property even where they suspect they will find evidence of ill-treatment. If they felt there were very strong grounds for suspicion, they might arrive with the police in the first place, or in extreme cases, where the end might be said to justify the means, they might possibly just enter anyway and hope that a court would be prepared to ignore what is in law a trespass if their suspicions are proved correct. The staff would not be trained to do this, but it is understandable how someone might take the decision to do it in the face of terrible suffering. The staff are not in any way a branch of the police, even though the RSPCA staff will have titles such as 'Inspector' or 'Superintendent', will be referred to as 'officers' and wear official looking uniforms. Staff from other welfare bodies may have a more informal approach. The police do have specific powers of arrest under the Protection of Animals Act 1911 and powers of entry under the Police and Criminal Evidence Act 1976.

You are not obliged to invite an RSPCA 'officer' onto your premises, nor do you have to say anything in answer to questions if you do not wish to. You may find that the 'officer' will adopt an official-type tone or mode of questioning, and you may be cautioned as you would be by a police officer to the effect that what you say may be used in evidence if a prosecution results, and that if you fail to say something at the point of initial questioning that you later use in your defence, the fact that you did not say it earlier may be questioned and harm the credibility of your defence. Watch out for not being cautioned at all. If you are not, then the welfare society may not be able to use anything you said in evidence.

If you are approached by an RSPCA official it should be made very clear to you that you are not under arrest; this can sometimes be misleading as it can give the impression that the 'officer' could arrest you if they wanted to but are not doing so at the moment. They may say they are just 'conducting enquiries' or 'looking into a complaint'. They will be unlikely to tell you where such a complaint has originated. You have to be careful not to inadvertently say something that might seem to incriminate you.

You can ask the 'officer' to leave your premises and he or she should do so. It is not recommended that any sort of physical contact is made or force used to get the 'officer' to leave. If you have nothing to hide and the 'officer' will not leave, then you could call the police yourself. But if you know any complaint is unfounded, why not just show the 'officer' around and reassure him or her? Sometimes the RSPCA do get malicious or misguided complaints, but it is in the interest of all animals that the complaints are investigated.

If they want to take matters further, they will need to enlist the help of the police. If the RSPCA 'officer' suspects there is a problem which has not been resolved by a visit and enquiries, he or she may caution you and then report the matter to the police, perhaps returning with them very soon after – they will not want to give you the opportunity to get rid of the evidence in the form of the ill-treated horse, or whatever. If the evidence is there you could be arrested, or taken to a police station for questioning. Your horse or horses could be seized by the police.

If you do have a genuine reason for having an apparently ill-treated animal on your premises, it might be as well to err on the side of caution and have evidence available to explain the problem. You might for instance have bought a horse in poor condition recently and be in the process of rehabilitating it, or your horse might have been extremely ill or is in the process of being investigated for a mystery illness. Many members of the public will not understand that a horse or pony prone to laminitis will need to be on very restricted grazing or even wear a muzzle, and they will complain of a pony being under-fed. (Do ensure that any horse or pony kept like this is monitored regularly and that the muzzle allows drinking and the escape of water from inside it.) Have a letter from your vet handy explaining the horse's health problems, or evidence of a recent purchase.

Prosecutions

If the RSPCA do decide to prosecute, it is most likely to be a 'private prosecution' brought by the Society itself, not by the police. If a case of cruelty is reported to the police, they will carry out the initial investigations and when they think they have enough evidence for a case to be brought, preferably for a conviction to be made, they will pass the matter to the Crown Prosecution Service (CPS) to do the actual court work and the hearings; or alternatively they will often pass it to the RSPCA because that organisation has considerable expertise in prosecuting cruelty claims and frequently has more experience and more access to suitably experienced lawyers than the police and the CPS. Any member of the public can attempt to prosecute someone privately for an offence, usually if the police cannot or will not, but it is quite difficult to do so as it will be expensive and time consuming. A private individual may also lack the investigative skills that the police have. However, the RSPCA do have funding and expertise and in many cases the police prefer to leave the prosecutions to them.

   If you do find yourself the subject of a possible prosecution, seek legal help as soon as possible. The Equine Lawyers Association has details of specialist solicitors who will defend people in this position. The RSPCA usually has a 'panel' of solicitors to choose from to do their legal work. Cruelty cases are unpopular and the tide of feeling will be against anyone even suspected of causing unnecessary suffering to an animal, however inadvertently. You may find that you need expert evidence if you know or feel you have a defence, and a specialist solicitor can help in finding a suitable expert. Although all cases should be defended where you feel the accusations are ill-founded and can probably be proved to be so, it may be all the more important when it is your business or reputation at stake. Local newspapers like few things better than a 'human interest' tale of suffering animals being rescued and given a happy ending, with the evil owners being given their just desserts – often quite rightly. Reporters are free to report any court case heard in open court unless the court imposes reporting restrictions, and you can guarantee that a cruelty case will be given some prominence.

Work of the International League for the Protection for Horses

Welfare organisations other than the RSPCA tend to work slightly differently and try to adopt a more persuasive approach in the hope that a cruel or hopeless owner will turn the horse over to them to be cared for or rehabilitated. As an example, the International League for the Protection of Horses (ILPH) fund a team of field officers, but like the RSPCA they have no specific policing or enforcement powers. The League was started in 1927 by Ada Cole to look into the welfare of horses being exported for slaughter. Despite some well-publicised problems, which still exist, there were relatively few complaints in this area and the League began to look at the rehabilitation and rehoming of horses, work which is now undertaken very widely. The League reports that cases of cruelty are evenly spread and no one area seems much worse than any other.

One of the problems with horse cruelty cases is that there are different classifications of horses; they can be agricultural or working animals or pet animals. Therefore it is difficult to make and enforce regulations that cover all horses, and there isn't one body responsible for their welfare.

The League works by identifying possible cruelty cases, either by complaints received from the public or the police, or from local knowledge of their field officers. They do have a system to try to identify malicious calls. If they feel there is a valid complaint, the field officer for that area will go and assess the situation and discuss and advise if allowed to. One of the biggest problems they encounter are situations where owners are clearly struggling to keep their horses – perhaps they have become unemployed, or have become ill and are encountering practical difficulties in looking after the horses. In these situations, the field officer might seek to persuade the owner to 'sign over' or gift the horse to the League for rehoming. In cases of convictions for cruelty, a court can order that this be done, but before that the officer has no power to take the horse if the owner will not agree. Therefore, many horses have to be left to deteriorate to the point where a cruelty prosecution can be brought and maintained, before anything can be done. If the officer finds clear evidence of cruelty at the time and the owner will not agree to sign over the horse, then the officer will call in the police. A vet will also need to be called as it is the vet who makes the decision as to whether the horse could be said to be 'suffering'. Neither the field officers nor the police make this judgement officially. The case will then continue in the usual way, with the police deciding whether there is enough evidence for the case to be referred to the CPS for possible prosecution.

The League have a policy of not buying horses; they believe this would lead to owners making money out of their own cruelty, so however distressing the situation they will not do it. They do rehome horses, vetting the applicants and new homes carefully and operating a monitoring system afterwards. They cannot make money from the horses, so cannot run riding schools or the like to make money, but they do accept donations and bequests, as do the RSPCA. Like the RSPCA they have a campaigning function, though they campaign only for horses, ponies and donkeys, whereas the RSPCA campaign for animal welfare generally.

Reporting cruelty

So what can you do if you suspect cruelty? Report it immediately. The societies will usually take anonymous phone calls if you are concerned about problems should the person you are complaining about get to know who made the complaint. Do not try to take any 'rescue' steps yourself, unless the situation is dire and requires immediate attention. No-one is going to criticise you for taking a bucket of water to a horse.

When reporting, give as much detail as you can. Do you know who the owner is? How long has the horse been subject to possible 'unnecessary suffering'? Do not report to different societies; this is confusing. Choose either a society or the police, though you will probably have more success with the societies unless you feel the situation is so serious that it justifies police intervention straight away, bearing in mind that the police do have the power to enter property and take animals into custody almost immediately. If one of the societies became involved, there might be a delay while they enlisted police support. You might find that you have to be convincing as to the urgency of the matter if you go straight to the police.

When you have reported to a society, make sure you contact them to check that your complaint has been investigated. Most will tell you the outcome; the ILPH has a positive policy of contacting the original complainant to tell them what has happened.

Don't make complaints maliciously or to cause trouble, but don't be afraid to make complaints. If you genuinely feel there is cause for concern, you could be saving a horse's life.

Chapter 19

The Final Parting with a Horse

What do you do when you realise, sadly, that your horse has come to the end of his life? You have decided that selling is not an option due to his age, illness or injury. He is not suitable as a loan companion and, anyway, you are worried that he will not really become a companion but will be sold on, and those you have loaned him to will disappear.

You could offer the horse to a rest home for retirement, but there are fewer and fewer of these. There may be private ones where you can pay for him to be cared for as he lives out the rest of his life, but ask yourself whether it is really worth it. If you have given him a happy life, could you not consider using the money to give a new horse the same chance? The BHS produce a leaflet *Caring For Old and Retired Horses*.

The good of the horse must always be the first consideration; so you take a deep breath and decide he has reached the end of his days. Remember to check your insurance policy to see if you need to inform your insurers before having your horse put down, otherwise any claim for loss may not be accepted. In an emergency, it is usually in order to inform the insurers as soon as possible afterwards.

Having the horse put down

Your options are:

- Your horse can be put down at home. This is likely to be the least traumatic for him. He can be buried at home if you have enough land and burial can be far enough away from certain facilities such as water courses. Check with the Department of the Environment, Food and Rural Affairs and your local Environmental Health Department as to whether you have a suitable and approved site. You may also need to contact the Environment Agency. You will need machinery capable of moving large quantities of earth, so even if you have a suitable site check that there is access. A vet will *have* to put down the horse if you want this to be by injection, but it would be usual in these situations for a vet to put him down whether by injection or humane killer.

- The horse can be put down at home and then transported to the knacker's yard. If you sell him or let him go to the knacker while still alive, he becomes the knacker's property. There have been cases where the knacker has patched up a horse and sold it on. If you have no other option, then consider going with your horse, however distressing, or if you really can't bear it try to get someone you trust to go with him and make sure he is put down. Knacker's yards are regulated and will almost certainly do a professional job, but you may want the peace of mind of knowing that the horse has really been put down. Knacker's yards generally produce meat for non-human or pet consumption, but there are EU approved yards that produce meat for human consumption. It is unlikely that you will want to use these.

- You can have the horse cremated. The crematorium will usually offer a complete service and can have the horse put down at your premises. This can be either by injection or humane killer. It will cost about £300–£500 if you have your horse cremated with others, and about £900 or more if you want him cremated alone so you can have the ashes. If you want to scatter the ashes, strictly speaking you may need permission from the local environmental health authority, but if you have enough of your own land there may be no problem. You can bury the ashes in a container in the ground, either at home or at the crematorium where there may be a Garden of Remembrance.

- You may want the local hunt to dispose of the horse and use him for hound food. This service is less common than it once was. In this situation, it is likely that the horse must be put down with a humane killer, as if he is put down by injection, he cannot enter the food chain for a certain period – check with your vet exactly what this period is. It is not only vets who can put horses down using a humane killer. Hunt staff are usually trained to do this and it is perfectly legal as long as there is no cruelty involved.

Making a will

Have you considered making a will? You cannot leave money to your horse as such, but if you have sufficient resources you can make financial provision for him to be looked after for his lifetime if you die before he does. This can be either by asking a welfare organisation to take him, along with enough money to keep him, or by giving him to a named and trusted individual. You should make sure that they are fully aware of your intentions before you do this. Not everyone wants to find themselves the unexpected owner of a large animal requiring a great deal of care, no matter how much money comes with it. South Essex Insurance Brokers have teamed up with Redwings Horse Sanctuary and offer a policy for horses over the age of 15 that will give a sum of money to the sanctuary at your death so that they can take your horse into their care.

You might also consider leaving a bequest to a horse charity. Many, if not all, rely heavily on gifts made by will for the finances to keep up their work, and they will be extremely grateful. Choose one or more whose aims you agree with and support, with alternatives in case the charity you choose ceases to exist.

If you do make a will, it is legal to draw up a home-made will or use a will form that can be bought from stationers, as long as either complies with the legal requirements for a will – but it is not recommended. Discuss your requirements with a specialist solicitor. You may think you don't have much in the way of assets to leave, but you may be surprised. Difficulties can arise later for families, if a will is unclear.

If you do not leave a will, particularly if you have no family or descendants to which to leave your estate, then you run the risk of your assets, including your horse or horses, being split up and sold, with the money going to those entitled to it by operation of law, rather than where you would have liked to see it go. In extreme cases, your money can go to the Crown when there is nowhere else for it to go. Wouldn't you rather see horses and ponies helped?

Appendix 1
Example Loan Agreement

This is an example of a loan agreement entered into by two imaginary parties, reflecting what they have agreed between them. Your own loan agreement may have different clauses and details. The important point is to draw up a document that both parties agree to and are happy to comply with. One party may have greater bargaining power than the other and there may have to be some element of compromise – it will depend on how much you want to loan or loan out this particular horse. If instinct tells you it really is not going to work – for instance as the loanee you find yourself in disagreement over almost everything the owner wants, or as the owner the loanee just doesn't seem knowledgeable enough – then it is probably best not to go ahead. Hopefully the process of trying to draw up a suitable agreement will expose any problems at an early stage.

This example is for guidance only. You are strongly advised to take independent legal advice before entering into any type of agreement or arrangement.

(*Text in italic indicates points to consider or alternatives.*)

Agreement for Loan of Horse

This Agreement is made between:

1. . . . .
   of . . . .

   ('the Owner')
   and

1. . . . .
   of . . . .

   ('the Loanee')

in respect of and in consideration of the loan by the Owner to the Loanee of the horse . . . . described below for the purpose of

. . . .

This Agreement is an Agreement for Loan and shall not be interpreted or construed as an Agreement for any other purpose.

The loan shall be for a period of . . . . ('the loan period'). *(Do you want an option for the loanee to renew? On the same or different terms? Do you want an option for the loanee to have first refusal if the horse is to be sold?)*

Prior to commencement of the loan period, there will be a probationary period of 28 days subject to the terms and conditions of this agreement and if after expiry of this probationary period, or earlier by mutual agreement of the Owner and the Loanee, the horse has proved suitable in the opinion of the Loanee, for the purpose of the loan, then the loan period will commence. *(You may not need this)*

If the horse does not prove suitable, in the Loanee's opinion, then the Loanee will return the horse to the Owner during the probationary period at his or her expense. *(Or at the Owner's expense, whichever is agreed).*

The Loanee's opinion will be final.

The *(here put in any other document which you want to become part of the terms of the Agreement)* . . . . shall form part of the Agreement.

The Probationary Period will commence on: . . . .

The Loan Period will commence on . . . .

The loan will terminate as follows:

     a) Upon either party giving … days notice in writing/by telephone to the other, such notice to take effect from the second day after the date of the notice if in writing or immediately if by telephone.

  or

     b) Immediately if either party is in breach of any of the terms and conditions of this agreement, save that if the breach is capable of remedy, either party can require the other to remedy any such breach by giving written notice of the breach, the action required to remedy it and the time by which the action must be performed. If the breach is so remedied, then the agreement will resume from that point.

  or

     c) At the end of the specified loan period if any without the need for any further notice.

or

    d) As may be specified in this agreement on the occurrence of a specific event.

The Loanee shall be responsible for transporting the horse back to the Owner on termination and for the costs involved however termination occurs.

or

Upon termination, under a) and d) the horse shall be removed by the Owner on the date specified in any notice or as set out in the Agreement or within 48 hours if under b) or c). If the horse is not so removed then the Loanee reserves the right to charge for livery at . . . . . per day, payable before the horse is removed.

The Horse *(Attach photos from front, back and both sides)*

Name: . . . .

Age: . . . .

Height: . . . .

Sex: . . . .

Breed: . . . .

Breed Reg. No: . . . .

Freeze mark: . . . .

Colour and description: . . . .

. . . .

. . . .

Any other identifying marks . . . .

. . . .

The horse . . . . known as ' . . . . ' is as described above and is warranted sound, free from any stable vices or other habits, good to box, shoe, clip, catch and in traffic, of good temperament to handle and ride and suitable for the purpose of the loan save as set out below:

. . . .

. . . .

. . . .

. . . .

The Owner warrants that he/she has hereby disclosed all known unsoundnesses, pre-existing health and/or dental conditions, vices, defects, habits or specific characteristics of the horse to the best of his/her knowledge and belief and the Loanee is taken to accept the horse with those so disclosed as above but with no other.

The Loanee reserves the right to require the Owner to remove the horse at any time at the Owner's expense should the horse prove not to be as described above and in particular if it is unsound, has one or more vices, is carrying any infectious disease or illness, or is, or becomes dangerous, in the opinion of the Loanee, to ride or handle.

Tack and Equipment

The horse is loaned with tack and equipment as set out below: *(Itemise each piece and give a description of it together with an agreed assessment of its condition. Attach photos if required.)*

. . . .
. . . .
. . . .
. . . .
. . . .
. . . .
. . . .
. . . .
. . . .
. . . .
. . . .

Such tack and equipment is and remains the property of the Owner and will be returned to the Owner at the termination of the loan in the same condition as far as possible, fair wear and tear excepted. Where return is not possible, due to loss, damage or the item wearing out, then a replacement item of the same or similar quality and value if purchased new should be provided by the Loanee on return. All additional items purchased by the Loanee during the period of the loan not by way of replacement shall remain the property of the Loanee. The Loanee will *not* insure any tack or equipment while it is in his/her possession under this agreement and if the Owner requires insurance cover for the tack and equipment then he/she *must* make their own arrangements, except that the Loanee will not be responsible for the provision or cost of any modifications to the premises where the horse is kept and/or systems necessary to comply with the terms of any policy and the cost of the same will be the responsibility of the Owner nor will the Loanee allow any modifications which in the Loanee's absolute discretion are deemed unreasonable and/or unreasonably required by the Owner even where this means that the terms of any policy cannot then be complied with.

For the avoidance of doubt, the Owner should obtain details of any policy requirements *before* taking out any policy and obtain express prior agreement to the terms of the policy from the Loanee.

The Loanee agrees with the Owner that in consideration of the Owner loaning the horse under this agreement he/she will:

1. Use the horse only for the purposes of the loan (*or* for the purpose of ...) and that the horse shall only be ridden and managed by . . . . *(and/or their agents or staff, and/or such outside instructors as shall be from time to time employed by the Loanee for teaching purposes. The horse will be used at the discretion of . . . ., but is unlikely to be required to work in excess of . . . . per day on . . . . days of the week. Consider competing – who gets the prize money, who pays for entry fees, etc., will the owner not want the horse taken beyond a certain level? If the purpose is for breeding, the terms of this agreement are unlikely to be suitable and a specific agreement should be drawn up. Is the Loanee willing to allow the owner to retain some riding rights? This can cause problems – what if both want to ride at the same time? What if the horse is injured while the owner is riding such that the loanee cannot use it for a considerable time? Who would pay for vet's bills in those circumstances? Could the Loanee terminate the loan?)*

2. Keep the horse at . . . . or such other premises as are appropriate at the discretion of the Loanee save that the Owner will be given ... days notice of any new address except in an emergency when the Owner will be notified as soon as possible.

3. Be responsible for all the horse's day to day care, including the provision of an adequate diet, stabling, bedding and grazing and take all reasonable care to maintain the horse in good condition, and for all costs involved in doing so. *(Specify any particular feed/bedding/other regimes if required. Who will be responsible for the cost of unusual or particularly expensive feed, supplements, bedding etc? Is the Loanee at liberty to change the horse's diet if he/she sees fit?)*

4. Have the horse regularly and appropriately shod by a suitably qualified farrier of the Loanee's choice at the Loanee's expense.

5. Keep the horse regularly and appropriately vaccinated and wormed according to the Loanee's programme and keep a record of the same, the cost of vaccinations and wormers to be met by the Loanee.

6. Ensure the provision of appropriate tack and equipment if not provided with the horse, at the Loanee's expense, but all and any such tack or equipment purchased by the Loanee for the horse shall remain

the property of the Loanee at all times and will not go with the horse on return. *(Consider whether the tack and equipment to be loaned with the horse is suitable, or whether the Loanee would prefer to buy their own in any case and keep it at the end of the loan period. Consider what to do about expensive items such as saddles, for example the Loanee will not want to return a nearly new £1500 dressage saddle as a replacement for an elderly general purpose saddle that came with the horse.)*

7. Provide proper and appropriate veterinary care and treatment by a veterinary surgeon and veterinary practice of the Loanee's choice as necessary on the following conditions:

   a) The Loanee will be responsible for the full cost of veterinary or dental treatment for any illness, injury or disease caused by the negligence of the Loanee during the period of the loan to the extent that it is not covered by insurance, provided that the treatment is recommended on veterinary advice by a veterinary surgeon retained by the Loanee.

   Where the veterinary advice is that the horse should be humanely destroyed whether on economic or humane grounds, then the Loanee reserves the right to refuse to meet the cost of any veterinary care or treatment beyond that advice and if the Owner wishes further treatment, then he/she must be responsible for the cost and for the cost of any livery, feed, bedding, shoes, wormer, vaccinations etc., whilst the horse is unfit for the purpose of the loan but still in the care of the Loanee. The Loanee shall not require any personal payment for his/her care of the horse during such time should it be the Loanee's decision to continue caring for the horse up to a period of . . . . but thereafter will require either that the horse be taken back by the Owner or that the Owner pay for the care of the horse at a rate of . . . . . . *(or whatever is the current livery rate at the time)* but for no longer than . . . . after which the horse must be taken back by the Owner.

   In the event of the horse's death while in the care of the Loanee, the Loanee will only offer compensation for the value of the horse where the horse is not insured for the same and where the horse's death has been caused by the Loanee's negligence and there is veterinary confirmation of that negligence. The amount of compensation will be the sum of . . . . agreed between the parties to this agreement *or* the value of the horse on the open market immediately prior to its death as evidenced and confirmed in writing by . . . . *(for instance, a reputable dealer in that type of animal or a reputable local dealer)*

b) The Loanee will otherwise be responsible for the cost of veterinary or dental care up to the value of £ . . . . for any illness, injury or disease not caused by the negligence of the Loanee where this is not covered by insurance during the period of the loan for any one incident but not for more than any . . . separate incidences in any . . . month period. Any costs over and above this sum must be borne by the Owner.

c) If the horse is diagnosed with an illness, disease or injury which is likely to be permanent or recurring on a regular basis and which is or is likely to render the horse unfit for the purpose of this loan then the Loanee reserves the right to return the horse to the Owner as soon as possible after such diagnosis and to require it to be moved from the Loanee's premises within . . . days of such diagnosis at the Owner's expense.

d) The Loanee will not meet the cost of veterinary or dental care and treatment for the pre-existing condition/s of . . . . *or* any pre-existing condition not disclosed to them by the Owner.

e) The Loanee will not meet the cost of veterinary or dental care where the veterinary or dental advice is that such treatment or care is uneconomic and/or unlikely to benefit the horse.

f) Although reasonable efforts will be made where possible to contact the Owner, the Loanee reserves the right to have the horse humanely destroyed or surgery performed on veterinary advice without obtaining the express prior permission of the Owner in an emergency and/or where the horse is suffering.

In non-emergency cases, where destruction or surgery is advised, reasonable efforts will be made to contact the Owner and obtain permission, but the Loanee reserves the right to have surgery performed and/or the horse destroyed after . . . . days or sooner on veterinary advice if the Owner cannot be contacted.

The Loanee will be responsible for the cost of disposal of the body should the horse be destroyed but reserves the right to do this by the most economic means. *(Otherwise note any specific requirements – e.g. cremation, putting down by injection and who will be responsible for the cost.)*

8. Be responsible for the horse's care while travelling during the period of the loan where this is arranged by the Loanee but will not be responsible for the horse's welfare to and from the Loanee at the start and termination of the loan period unless specifically organised by the Loanee nor while the horse is being transported under arrangements made by the Owner.

9. Allow the Owner access at all reasonable times to the horse on the Owner giving at least . . . hours notice to . . . .

10. Not sell, attempt to sell or enter into any agreement to sell the horse during the period of the loan, nor loan the horse to any other person or persons, authorities or bodies without the prior written permission and the full knowledge of the Owner.

11. At all times treat the horse with patience and kindness and not require it to perform beyond its reasonable capabilities in the discretion of the Loanee.

And the Owner agrees that in consideration of the same, he/she will:

1. Accept the terms of and the responsibilities, financial or otherwise, as set out in this Agreement.

2. *(Any other specific responsibilities of the Owner if not mentioned under any other heading.)*

3. Give the Loanee quiet enjoyment of the horse under this Agreement.

Arbitration

The Loanee and the Owner agree that any disputes or complaints arising with regard to the horse during the period of the loan whether arising out of the terms and conditions of this agreement or otherwise which cannot be resolved to both parties' satisfaction by first raising the matter with . . . . in writing within . . . . days of the dispute or complaints arising, specifying the grounds of the dispute or complaint and specifying the remedy required, shall be referred to . . . .

(nominated by the party requesting arbitration. If the other party objects, he or she must do so in writing within 7 days of being notified either by telephone or in writing of the nomination or the nomination stands. If an arbitrator is not agreed an arbitrator shall be appointed by ....) as sole arbitrator(s) for arbitration and decision, such decision to be accepted as final and binding by and on both parties.

The arbitrator's fees and expenses shall be borne in equal shares by the parties who shall have no other claim against each other whatsoever in respect of those fees or expenses, otherwise each party shall be responsible for their own costs of such arbitration and decision.

N.B. You may lose your right to take Court action by agreeing to Arbitration

We understand and agree to the terms and conditions of this loan agreement as set out above and agree that it contains the entire terms of the agreement, superseding and replacing any prior oral or written communications between the Loanee and the Owner.

(Witnesses should be independent and unconnected to the Agreement.)

Signed .... Owner   Print name ....
Dated ....

Witnessed ....   Print name ....
Dated ....   Address ....

Witnessed ....   Print name ....
Dated ....   Address ....

Signed .... Loanee   Print name ....
Dated ....

Witnessed ....   Print name ....
Dated ....   Address ....

Witnessed ....   Print name ....
Dated ....   Address ....

Disclaimer

Neither Brenda Gilligan nor Pritchard Englefield, Solicitors, or their employees, servants or agents, or anyone acting, purporting to act or holding themselves out as acting for either, can be responsible for any loss or damage, financial or otherwise, or injury, or any other adverse outcome howsoever caused, as a result of use of this sample loan agreement where the user has not taken independent legal advice on the contents of their own specific loan agreement prior to entering into any agreement or other arrangement, whether for loan or otherwise. It is strongly advised that you take such advice before entering into any type of agreement or arrangement, whether for a loan or otherwise. This sample is for guidance only.

Appendix 2
Example Full Livery Agreement

This is an example livery agreement only. Ensure that your own livery agreement reflects your personal requirements and that you are happy to comply with its terms.

Full Livery Agreement

This agreement is made between:

1. **Hill Top Equestrian Centre, High Street, Yelling, Cambridgeshire**

('Hill Top')

and

2. . . . .

of . . . .

('the Livery')

This Agreement is an Agreement for Full Livery of the horse or horses belonging to or in the care of the Livery as set out in the annexed Schedule 1 and shall not be interpreted or construed as an Agreement for any other purpose.

The Livery agrees to abide by the conditions of this Agreement and any other reasonable rules, regulations, terms, conditions and the like that may be from time to time required by Hill Top, including all Health and Safety regulations and/or legal requirements which must be fulfilled by Hill Top. Notice of these are currently posted at . . . . and the Livery's attention is hereby drawn to them.

Under this agreement, the Livery agrees to pay a livery fee of . . . . . per horse every 4 weeks, due and payable 4 weeks in advance. The livery fee will be reviewed annually on the . . . . and may be subject to increase of which 4 weeks' notice will be given.

The livery period is subject to a 4 week probationary period commencing on . . . . and ending on . . . . 4 weeks notice from either party is required to be given in writing in order to bring the livery period to an end except where otherwise stated in this Agreement. Hill Top also reserve the right to terminate this Agreement immediately where the terms of this Agreement have been breached by the Livery and not rectified within 14 days of being asked to do so, or in cases of cruelty to any animal whether belonging to the Livery or not, verbal or physical abuse of any person or animal, theft or dishonesty by the Livery or anyone acting on their behalf.

In consideration of this and provided the conditions of this Agreement are kept, Hill Top will provide full livery services to the Livery as follows:

1. Stables

- All horses are kept on shavings, which will be provided by Hill Top to the extent of two bales of shavings per week. If the livery requires special shavings, i.e. dust extracted, or more than two bales per week, then these will have to be provided by the Livery at their own expense.

- Daily mucking out and skipping out of the horse's stable to a clean condition and weekly clearance of all wet shavings.

- Hill Top will provide and maintain the stable allocated to the horse(s) but any damage caused by the Livery's horse must be repaired to a good standard by the Livery at his or her expense as soon as possible after the damage has occurred and at the latest 14 days after the damage provided that the damage is not presenting a danger to any person or animal likely to be present on the yard. Hill Top reserve the right to repair the damage themselves and to bill the Livery for work and materials. Where a horse continually damages stables then the Livery may be asked to consider keeping the horse at grass if this would be available at the discretion of Hill Top, but where this is not an option then the Livery may be asked to move. Hill Top cannot guarantee that any particular stable will be available and the Livery may be required to move stables where necessary.

2. Feeding

- Feed will be provided to the extent of two feeds per day given at approximately 8–9AM and 4–5PM fed at the rate of . . . . or at the discretion of Hill Top as appropriate, using Alfa-A, Jordan's 12% coarse mix and sugar beet, unless alternative arrangements are agreed. If the horse(s) require(s) extra or different feed, supplements or additives, these will have to be supplied at the Livery's own expense and full details of feeding regime are to be supplied to Hill

Top. If the Livery requires the horse to be fed at a different time, i.e. due to show commitments, then 48 hours' notice is to be given, except that Hill Top will not be able to be responsible for feeds to be given before 7AM or after 8PM and the Livery must in those cases make their own arrangements including arranging access to the yard and feed rooms with Hill Top.

- Hay or horsehage/haylage is provided in the discretion of Hill Top appropriate to each individual horse's requirements divided into two nets given one in the morning and one in the evening. The Livery must provide two small-hole hay nets and replace as necessary. If anything other than hay or horsehage/haylage is required this must be provided by the Livery at his or her own expense.

3. Water

- Water is provided by Hill Top, but care is required not to waste water or use water unnecessarily as the water is metered. Livery to provide at least two heavy duty water buckets for stable.

4. Fields and Grazing

- Fields, grazing and fencing (including electric fencing) will be provided and maintained by Hill Top. Water will be provided by Hill Top for the fields. Livery to provide at least one good quality head-collar and lead rope. Livery to state whether to be left on or off whilst out. On/Off

- Horses will be turned out daily where possible providing weather conditions are suitable. The decision on this will be made by Hill Top. Winter turnout will be restricted to small winter paddocks which are liable to become muddy, or into the arena for up to one hour only per day.

- In summer, horses can be turned out all day and night provided this is appropriate for the horse and there is space, but there will be no reduction in livery cost if this is required.

- In any event horses will be left out as long as possible and can be brought in by the Livery or by arrangement with Hill Top. Hill Top will in any case bring in horses at their discretion where appropriate.

- Horses are turned out in groups of mares and geldings where possible. The Livery will be responsible for ensuring that their horse(s) is/are safe to turn out with other horses and if they are not then Hill Top should be notified prior to the commencement of the livery agreement as it may not be possible to accommodate such horses. Any special requirements should be discussed with Hill Top prior to commencement of the livery agreement.

- Horses' legs will be washed off where necessary on being brought in.

5. Arena

- The Livery is entitled to use of the arena but must exercise consideration to other riders already in the arena or wishing to use the arena. The arena may be used during private lessons subject to the discretion of the instructor.

- Hill Top will be responsible for the lights in the arena but in winter (between . . . . and . . . .) use of the arena lights will not be allowed before . . . . or after . . . .

- When using the arena all care must be taken to use the arena safely and proper and appropriate equipment must be used. When riding or lungeing, an approved safety riding hat or skull cap must be worn together with proper riding boots. Hill Top recommend gloves are worn when lungeing.

- Other riders must be warned before entering and leaving the arena. The arena gate must be closed when the arena is in use.

- Horses' feet must be clean before entering the arena and must be picked out after leaving the arena into the skip, provided.

- All droppings must be cleared.

- Jumps, trotting poles etc. must be put away after use unless specifically required by another rider.

6. Yard

- All areas of the yard must be left in a clean and tidy state with all droppings cleared up, the area in front of the Livery's stable swept and all belongings put away.

- All belongings and equipment must be clearly labelled and kept tidily. You should not use anyone else's equipment without their express permission and all equipment must be returned promptly if borrowed.

- Tack must not be left at the yard unless Hill Top are responsible for exercising your horse in which case it will be kept at the main house, but no responsibility can be taken for loss or damage.

- Horses' feet must be picked out before leaving the stable to avoid shavings on the yard.

- The yard gate must remain closed at all times.

7. Rugs

- The Livery is responsible for the provision and maintenance of suitable summer, winter and stable rugs where used.

- Hill Top will be responsible for putting on and taking off rugs where they are responsible for putting the horses in and out but not otherwise.

8. Worming

- On arrival, new horses must be wormed using the appropriate product for the time of year and kept in for 24 hours thereafter.

- After the initial worming. Hill Top then have a worming programme for the whole yard which must be followed. Wormer can be supplied by Hill Top at cost to the Livery but will require 1 week's notice prior to worming date together with the cost of the wormer to enable ordering. Alternatively, the Livery can supply the wormer but it must be the same product as used by the yard. If the Livery has neither ordered nor provided wormer at the time worming is due, Hill Top reserve the right to worm the horse(s) nonetheless and charge the owner accordingly.

9. Shoeing

- All horses must be appropriately shod or have their feet trimmed every 6 weeks or as advised by a qualified and registered farrier.

- Hill Top have a farrier call regularly, but the Livery may use an alternative qualified and registered farrier if required. In either case, the farrier can be paid direct by the Livery, or the farrier's fee can be left with Hill Top to pass on. If no money is left to pay the farrier, the horse will not be shod or trimmed.

- All horses must be fully insured and a copy of the insurance certificate lodged with Hill Top. It is the responsibility of the Livery to ensure that all terms and conditions of the insurance policy are met and complied with and receipt of the copy policy does not imply that Hill Top have any notice of the terms and conditions of the policy nor that they will take steps to comply with them. It is the Livery's responsibility to bring any particular term or condition to the attention of Hill

Top where this may require Hill Top to take any actions. For the avoidance of doubt, the Livery should check the terms and conditions of any insurance policy before entering into it to ensure that they can comply with them.

10. Inoculations

- All horses must be fully inoculated at least against influenza and tetanus and it will be the responsibility of the Livery to ensure that these are kept up to date.

- All horses must be registered with a suitable veterinary practice and the name, address and telephone numbers of the vet lodged with Hill Top. It is the Livery's responsibility to ensure that the horse(s) receive proper veterinary and dental care.

- Hill Top reserve the right to call out a vet of their choice at their discretion where necessary, particularly in cases of severe illness, injury, infections, or suffering, but responsibility for the fees will be the Livery's. In emergency situations or on veterinary advice, although all reasonable efforts will be made to contact the Livery first, Hill Top reserve the right to authorise surgery and/or the humane destruction and disposal of the horse(s) by cremation whether or not this complies with insurance requirements. The fees will be the responsibility of the Livery.

11. General

- Where any fees, bills or invoices, whether rendered by Hill Top or otherwise are due and payable, these must be paid within 7 days of the date of the fee note, bill or invoice or as requested by the sender of it. Where there is persistent failure to pay monies owing in the discretion of Hill Top, the livery agreement will be terminated on 7 days' notice.

- While every reasonable care will be taken, neither Hill Top, nor any of its employees or staff, servants or agents, will be responsible for any loss, damage, injury or death of any person, animal or object, howsoever caused save for their liabilities in English Law.

- Hill Top will not be responsible in any way for the actions of any of their pupils even where this results in loss, damage, injury or death to the Livery. It will be the Livery's responsibility to take up any cause of action with the person concerned individually.

- Schedules 1, 2 and 3 annexed form part of this Agreement

12. Arbitration

- Hill Top and the Livery agree that any disputes or complaints arising with regard to the terms and conditions of this Agreement or in the way in which the terms and conditions have been interpreted or carried out should first try to be resolved by the complainant first raising the matter with . . . . in writing within . . . . . . days of the dispute or complaint arising, specifying the grounds of the dispute or complaint and specifying the remedy required.

- If the matter cannot be resolved in this way, then it shall be referred to an independent veterinary surgeon or an independent Fellow of the British Horse Society (whichever is more appropriate) nominated by the British Horse Society at both parties' request to act as arbitrator. Such referral shall be made within 14 days of the dispute or complaint remaining unresolved.

- The arbitrator's decision will be final and binding and both parties agree to accept and abide by the arbitrator's decision.

- The arbitrator's fees and expenses shall be borne in equal shares by the parties who shall have no further claim against each other whatsoever in respect of those fees or expenses, otherwise each party shall be responsible for their own costs of such arbitration and decision.

We understand and agree to the terms and conditions of the livery Agreement as set out above and that it replaces and supersedes any previous agreements whether made orally or in writing whether by Hill Top, its employees or staff, servants or agents or anyone acting or claiming to act on its behalf.

Signed . . . .
Dated . . . .

For and on behalf of Hill Top Equestrian Centre

Signed . . . .
Dated . . . .

Livery/authorised to sign for and on behalf of Livery

Schedule 1

The Horse

Name: . . . .
Age: . . . .
Height: . . . .
Sex: . . . .
Breed: . . . .
Breed Reg. No: . . . .
Freeze mark: . . . .
Colour and Description: . . . .
. . . .
. . . .

The horse . . . . known as '. . . . .' is as described above and is sound, free from any stable vices or other habits, good to box, shoe, clip, catch and in traffic, of good temperament to handle and ride save as set out below:
. . . .
. . . .
. . . .
. . . .
. . . .

The Livery confirms that he/she has hereby disclosed all known unsoundness, pre-existing health and/or dental conditions or problems, vices, defects, habits or specific characteristics of the horse to the best of his/her knowledge and belief and Hill Top is taken to accept the horse with those so disclosed as above but with no other.

Hill Top reserve the right to require the Livery to remove the horse immediately at any time at the Livery's expense should the horse prove not to be as described above and in particular if it is has one or more vices likely to affect other horses on the yard detrimentally, is carrying any infectious disease or illness, or is, or becomes dangerous, in the opinion of Hill Top, to ride or handle.

Schedule 2

Tack and Equipment

The horse is liveried with tack and equipment as set out below:

. . . .
. . . .
. . . .
. . . .
. . . .
. . . .
. . . .
. . . .
. . . .

Hill Top will be responsible for cleaning of all tack and equipment, but not for repair, replacement or upkeep. It is the Livery's responsibility to keep the tack and equipment in a safe condition.

Tack and equipment is and remains the property of the Livery. Hill Top will *not* insure any tack or equipment whilst it is in their possession under this agreement and if the Livery requires insurance cover for the tack and equipment then he/she *must* make their own arrangements, except that Hill Top will not be responsible for the provision or cost of any modifications to its premises and/or systems necessary to comply with the terms of any policy, such modifications and the cost of the same will be the responsibility of the Livery nor will Hill Top allow any modifications which in Hill Top's absolute discretion are deemed to be unreasonable and/or unreasonably required by the Livery even where this means the terms of any policy cannot then be complied with.

For the avoidance of doubt, the Livery should obtain details of any policy requirements before taking out any policy and obtain express prior permission to the terms of the policy from Hill Top where necessary.

Schedule 3

Optional extras

Hill Top will not be responsible for the following unless specifically requested when such services can be provided at the cost stated, such costs to be reviewed annually on the ....

1. Grooming	Daily grooming included in cost of Full Livery.
2. Exercising	Sharon: £10.00 per horse per session _____ up to 1 hour.
	Staff: £5.00 per horse per session _____ up to 1 hour.
3. Lungeing	Sharon: £10.00 per horse per session _____ up to 1 hour.
	Staff: £5.00 per horse per session _____ up to 1 hour.
4. Tack cleaning	£5.00 per saddle and bridle. £1.50 per_____ piece after that.
5. Show preparation	Bathing, mane and tail plaited. £35.00_____ per horse. 7 days notice usually required.
6. Clipping	Between £15.00 and £40.00 per horse _____ depending on clip. Horse must be good to clip. £15.00 extra charge if difficult horse.

Please tick if required on a regular basis and set out beside the service the agreed terms, e.g. 'once a week', 'each time used' etc.

Appendix 3

Sample of Certificate of Veterinary Examination

CERTIFICATE No:
V 02277

This is to certify that, at the request of (Name & Address) _____

I have examined the horse described below, the property of (Name & Address) _____

at (Place of Examination) _____ on (Time & Date) _____

NAME of horse (or breeding)	**INSTRUCTIONS** 1) WRITTEN DESCRIPTION SHOULD BE TYPED OR WRITTEN IN BLOCK CAPITALS 2) WRITTEN DESCRIPTION AND DIAGRAM SHOULD AGREE 3) ALL WHITE MARKINGS SHOULD BE HATCHED IN RED 4) WHORLS MUST BE SHOWN THUS "X" AND DESCRIBED IN DETAIL
BREED OR TYPE	
COLOUR	
SEX	
AGE by documentation	
APPROX. AGE by dentition **(See Note 1 - overleaf)**	

LEFT SIDE   RIGHT SIDE

FORE REAR VIEW   HIND REAR VIEW

HEAD AND NECK VENTRAL VIEW   MUZZLE   LEFT   RIGHT   LEFT   RIGHT

IDENTIFICATION

Head: _____

Neck: _____

Limbs: LF _____

RF _____

LH _____

RH _____

Body: _____

Acquired marks/brands/microchip: _____

REPORT OF EXAMINATION (See Note 2): I find no clinically discoverable signs of disease, injury or physical abnormality other than those here recorded (or recorded on the attached sheet)

_____

Cont'd on attached sheet Yes/No

Radiological or specialised techniques included in addition to the standard procedure _____

Report appended YES/NO   Blood taken and stored for testing for NSAIDs and other substances YES/NO   **WARRANTY (see Note3)**

THE OPINION (See Note 4): <u>On the balance of probabilities the conditions set out above</u> | **ARE** | **ARE NOT** | Delete clearly as appropriate

<u>likely to prejudice this animal's use for</u> _____

Owing to _____ stages _____ of the standard procedure were omitted **(See Note 5)**

Veterinary Surgeon's Signature _____ Date of Signature _____

Veterinary Surgeon's Name (in block capitals) _____

Address _____

NOTES - See overleaf

225

NOTE 1 - AGE:

Estimates of age based on an examination of dentition are imprecise and unreliable. In my opinion the approximate age is as stated and/or within the range shown. If the term 'aged' is used, this means that in my opinion the animal is over 8 years old.

NOTE 2 - THE EXAMINATION:

This clinical examination was carried out substantially in accordance with the standard procedure recommended by the RCVS/BVA Joint Memorandum on the Examination of Horses 1976 (revised 1986). The examination was conducted in five stages.

1.   Preliminary Examination
2.   Trotting up
3.   Strenuous exercise
4.   Period of rest
5.   A second trot up and foot examination

(All stages are usually carried out but if, for any reason, any stage is missed the opinions expressed are based on that restricted examination. It should be clear on the certificate overleaf in what way the examination has been varied).

NOTE 3 - WARRANTY:

If purchasers wish to obtain a warranty covering such matters as height, freedom from vices, temperament, the non-administration of drugs prior to examination or the animal's existing performance as a hunter, show-jumper, riding pony, eventer, etc., they are advised to seek such warranty in writing from the vendor, as these are matters between vendor and purchaser and are not the responsibility of the veterinary surgeon.

This certificate does not cover an examination for pregnancy.

NOTE 4 - OPINION:

The opinion expressed overleaf is based solely on the clinical examination set out above and is given subject to the qualification that the said animal may be presently subject to some previously administered drug or medicament intended to or having the effect of masking or concealing some disease, injury or physical abnormality which might otherwise presently be clinically discoverable.

NOTE 5 - REF. STAGES OMITTED:

My opinion is based on a partial examination only and does not establish any clinical signs of disease, injury or abnormality which would have manifested themselves only in the course of that part, or those parts, of the standard procedure which was, or were, omitted.

Appendix 4
Driver Licensing Requirements for Towing Trailers

(Reproduced by kind permission of the British Horse Society)

Changes in entitlement to tow trailers to comply with EC Directive on the Driving Licence

These changes came into effect on 1 January 1997 and affect all drivers having passed their test after that date and some existing drivers.

All **drivers who passed their test** *before* **1 January 1997** will not be affected by these changes, therefore retaining their existing entitlement to tow trailers, *except* for holders of category C (Lorries) or D (Buses) entitlement who wish to haul large trailers.

Car **drivers having obtained their full driving licence** *before* **1 January 1997**, are generally entitled to drive vehicles within the following categories:

- B   Vehicles up to 3.5 tonnes and with up to 8 passenger seats

- B+ E   As above + large trailer (over 750 kg)

- C1   Medium sized goods vehicles (3.5–7.5 tonnes) e.g. horse box

- C1 + E As C1 above + large trailer (over 750 kg) which allows vehicle and trailer combinations up to 8.5 tonnes to be driven.

However, **drivers having passed their driving test** *after* **1 January 1997 (new drivers)**, need to pass additional tests for each category in order to gain equivalent entitlement. The following information outlines the new drivers' entitlements, and which additional tests are necessary.

Category B: Vehicles up to 3.5 tonnes

A **new** driver may drive: 3.5 tonne vehicle + 750 kg trailer.
Category B vehicle (< 3.5 tonnes) + large trailer provided combination does not exceed 3.5 tonnes and the laden weight of the trailer does not

exceed the unladen weight of the towing vehicle. Thus the heavier the car, the heavier the trailer which may be towed, subject to the 3.5 tonne limit.

But **drivers of heavier vehicles towing larger trailers**, such as a laden horse-trailer, would need to take a further test for Category B + E.

NB: An exemption from the trailer limit will be introduced to allow a category B licence holder to tow a broken down vehicle from a position where it would otherwise cause danger or obstruction to other road users.

Category B + E: Vehicles up to 3.5 tonnes with large trailer

Heavy vehicles towing large horse-trailers would fall into this category. The EC Directive does not set an upper weight limit for this category, although Construction and Use Regulations limit the laden weight of unbraked trailers to no more than half the unladen weight of the towing vehicle. However, there is no specific limit for braked trailers.

Sub-category C1: Medium sized goods vehicles 3.5–7.5 tonnes

In order to gain the entitlement to drive sub-category C1 vehicles e.g. non-HGV horse boxes, a new driver with a standard licence (category B) will have to pass an additional test, as well as meet the higher medical standards required, which presently apply to all bus or lorry drivers.

C1 vehicles may be coupled with a trailer weighing up to 750 kg, but this trailer weight is an absolute limit.

Sub-category C1 + E: Medium sized goods vehicles with large trailer

This category allows vehicles to be coupled with a trailer over 750 kg, provided the combination does not exceed 12 tonnes and the laden weight of the trailer does not exceed the unladen weight of the towing vehicle.

New drivers would have to pass two further tests to gain this entitlement: C1 followed by C1 + E.

EC regulations limit **drivers under 21** to vehicles and combinations which weigh no more than 7.5 tonnes. **18 year olds** can take a test for category C1 + E allowing trailers in excess of 750 kg to be towed but they will be restricted to drive a combination weight of 7.5 tonnes until age 21 years when entitlement to drive up to 12 tonnes becomes automatic.

Category C: Large goods vehicles above 3.5 tonnes

These vehicles e.g. HGV horse boxes, may be combined with a trailer up to 750 kg. New drivers with a standard (category B) licence will have to pass a further test for category C. (It is not necessary to first gain sub-category C1 entitlement).

Category C + E: Large goods vehicles over 3.5 tonnes with trailer over 750 kg

In order to gain this entitlement, new drivers with a standard (category B) licence will have to pass two further tests – category C followed by category C + E.

Provisional trailer entitlement issued before 1 January 1997

As of 1 January 1997 it is no longer possible to sit a test in a heavy vehicle/ trailer combination (e.g. category C + E or D + E) unless a test in the corresponding rigid vehicle (e.g. category C or D) has been passed.

This means that although a driver may have been driving a vehicle and trailer combination legitimately under L plates, he/she is not permitted to sit a trailer test using such a combination until he/she has passed a test in a solo vehicle.

Maximum authorised mass (MAM)

Maximum authorised mass of vehicles and trailers means the permissible maximum weight, i.e. gross vehicle weight.

Manufacturer's weight recommendations as relates to insurance

Some confusion has risen from this new legislation with regard to weight ratios when towing. Drivers having obtained their full car driving licence before 1 January 1997 retain their entitlement. However, exceeding the manufacturer's maximum towing or maximum train weight, while not an offence in itself, may render the driver liable to prosecution for driving a dangerous vehicle and may invalidate insurance cover. Drivers are advised to check with their insurers that they have appropriate cover.

LPB/DVB/RS/01/49
30 January 1998

Appendix 5
Claim Form

This is the legal document that will begin your case formally when issued.

Claim Form

In the Cambridge County Court
Claim No.

Claimant

SEAL

Defendant(s)

Brief details of claim

Value

		£
Defendant's name and address	Amount claimed	
	Court fee	
	Solicitor's costs	
	Total amount	
	Issue date	

The court office at Bridge House

is open between 10 am and 4 pm Monday to Friday. When corresponding with the court, please address forms or letters to the Court Manager and quote the claim number.

N1 Claim form (CPR Part 7) (10.00)   Laserform International 09/00

Claim No.	

Does, or will, your claim include any issues under the Human Rights Act 1998?   ☐ Yes   ☐ No

Particulars of Claim (attached) (to follow)

Statement of Truth
* (I believe) (The Claimant believes)   that the facts stated in these particulars of claim are true.
* I am duly authorised by the claimant to sign this statement

Full name _____

Name of claimant's solicitor's firm   Pritchard Englefield _____

signed _____   position or office held _____
*(Claimant) (Litigation friend) (Claimant's solicitor)   (if signing on behalf of firm or company)

*delete as appropriate

Pritchard Englefield
14 New Street
London
EC2M 4HE

DX88   London

Claimant's or claimant's solicitor's address to
which documents or payments should be sent if
different from overleaf including (if appropriate)
details of DX, fax or e-mail.

Appendix 6
Useful Addresses

Association of British Riding
  Schools
Queens Chambers
38–40 Queen Street
Penzance
Cornwall TR18 4BH
Tel: 01736 369440
Fax: 01736 351390
e-mail: officer@abrs.org

Promotion of the provision of good
riding facilities and instruction for
the general public through an
approval and membership scheme
for riding establishments.

Association of Chartered
  Physiotherapists in Animal
  Therapy
Morland House
Salters Lane
Winchester
Hampshire
SO22 5JP
Tel: 01962 863801

British Association of Equine
  Dental Technicians
Mary-Lou Lees
The Bungalow
Bonehill Road
Mile Oak
Tamworth
Staffordshire
B78 3PS
Tel: 01827 284718
e-mail: mllees@dircom.co.uk

Umbrella organisation for equine
dental technicians, with
registration and regulation of
technicians.

British Association of
  Homeopathic Veterinary
  Surgeons
Chinham House
Stanford-in-the-Vale
Oxfordshire
SN7 8NQ
Tel: 01367 710324

British Equestrian Directory
Wothersome Grange
Bramham
Nr Wetherby
West Yorkshire
LS23 6LY
Tel: 0113 289 2267
e-mail: bed@emc.u-net.com
www.beta-uk.org

Comprehensive annual directory
of names, addresses and contact
details for all things equestrian.

British Equine Veterinary
    Association
5 Finlay Street
London SW6 6HE
Tel: 020 7610 6080
Fax: 020 7610 6823
e-mail: bevauk@msn.com

Association and forum for vets and
others with an interest in equine
veterinary science. Promotion of
and research into veterinary and
allied sciences related to equine
disorders and the welfare of the
horse.

British Equestrian Insurance
    Brokers Limited
Hildenbrook House
The Slade
Tonbridge
Kent TN9 1HR
Tel: 01732 771719

Only independent equestrian
Lloyds insurance brokers. Provides
impartial advice and provision of
equine insurance needs.

British Horse Society
Stoneleigh Deer Park
Kenilworth
Warwickshire CV8 2XZ
Tel: 08707 202 244
www.bhs.org.uk/

Charity and main source of
information on all things
equestrian and equine. Approval
scheme for riding establishments,
and register of instructors and
riding clubs.

Country Land and Business
    Association
16 Belgrave Square
London SW1X 8PQ
Tel: 020 7235 0511
Fax: 020 7235 4696
www.cla.org.uk

Association for anyone interested
in the country and rural affairs,
whether land-owners or not.
Publishes a regular journal, leaflets
and books on rural matters. Holds
an annual game fair, provides
information, education and
participates in campaigning.
Membership includes access to free
legal advice.

Department of the Environment,
    Food and Rural Affairs (DEFRA)
Tel: 0117 372 8957 – Countryside
    Division
www.defra.gov.uk

Government department now responsible for bridleways and country matters. Has taken over much of the functions of DETR (Department for Transport, Environment and the Regions) and MAFF (Ministry of Agriculture, Fisheries and Food).

Department of Trade and Industry
Tel:: 0845 6000 678
www.dti.gov.uk/er/nmw
www.tiger.gov.uk (specifically
   minimum wage rates)

Starting point for workplace information for employers and employees.

Equine Lawyers Association
P. O. Box 23
Brigg
Lincolnshire DN20 8TN
Tel: 01652 688819

http://members.aol.com/ukbiz/
peachey.htm

Association of lawyers interested in and with expertise in all aspects of equine law. Publisher of *Horse Law* journal.

Farriers Registration Council
Sefton House
Adams Court
Newark Road
Peterborough
PE1 5PP
Tel: 01733 319911
www.farrier-reg.gov.uk

Regulation and registration of farriers.

Health and Safety Executive
RIDDOR (Reporting of Injuries,
   Diseases and Dangerous
   Occurrences Regulations 1995)
Incident Contact Centre
Caerphilly Business Park
Caerphilly
CF83 3GG
Tel: 0845 300 9923
Fax: 0845 300 9924
HSE info line: 0870 1545500
HSE information centre e-mail:
hseinformationservices@
   natbrit.com
RIDDOR e-mail:
   riddor@natbrit.com
www.riddor.gov.uk,
www.hse.gov.uk

Centre for reporting of accidents at work or otherwise under the regulations, plus information on health and safety laws and regulations.

Horse and Hound
www.horseandhound.co.uk

Website of the popular equestrian weekly magazine. News and information over a wide area of equestrian disciplines, horses and equipment for sale, competition and show reports and results, racing, hunting and much more.

Ifor Williams Trailers Limited
www.iwt.co.uk

Information on trailers, towing and training.

International League for the
Protection of Horses
Anne Colvin House
Hall Farm
Snetterton
Norwich
Norfolk NR16 2LR
Tel: 01953 498682
Fax: 01953 498373

Charity concerned with the welfare
of horse, ponies and donkeys,
including rehabilitation and
rehoming of equines. Team of field
officers. Education, campaigning
and fundraising.

International Spinal Research Trust
Bramley Business Centre
Station Road
Bramley
Guildford
Surrey
GU5 0AZ
Tel: 01483 898 786
Fax: 01483 898 763
e-mail: isrt@spinal-research.org
www.spinal-research.org

Research into spinal injuries

The Law Society
113 Chancery Lane
London WC2A 1PL
Tel: 020 7242 1222
www.lawsociety.co.uk

Solicitors' professional association
and governing body, with database
of specialist lawyers in all areas of
law.

Local Ombudsman
21 Queen Anne's Gate
London
SW1H 9BU

Resolution of complaints with
regard to procedures of local
authority bodies, i.e. delay.

Mark Davies Injured Riders Fund
Little Woolpit
Ewhurst
Cranleigh
Surrey GU6 7NP
Tel: 01258 817859
www.mdirf.co.uk

Charity supporting those injured in
equestrian accidents with advice
and financial help, plus research
into horse and rider safety.

Medical Equestrian Association
The Medical Commission of
Accident Prevention
C/o 35–43 Lincolns Inn Fields
London
WC2A 3PN
Tel: 020 7242 3176

Association of medics and other
parties interested in horse and
rider safety, improving safety
standards and the provision and
standard of medical treatment for
riders.

National Equine Welfare Council
Stanton
10 Wales Street
King's Sutton
Nr Banbury
Oxon
OX17 3RR
Tel/Fax: 01295 810 060
e-mail:
  newckingssutton@freeserve.co.uk

National Trailer and Towing
  Association Limited
1 Alveston Place
Leamington Spa
Warwickshire
CV32 4SN
Tel: 01926 335445
e-mail: info@ntta.co.uk
www.ntta.co.uk

Trade association covering every
aspect of the light trailer industry,
with help, advice and information
for trade and public on towing law,
trailers and towing vehicles.

Organisation of Horsebox and
  Trailer Owners
Whitehill Farm
Hamstead Marshall
Newbury
Berkshire
RG20 0ZZ
Tel: 01488 657651

Specialist recovery schemes for box
and trailer owners.

Peaceful Pets
West Rudham
King's Lynn
Norfolk
PE31 8SY
Tel: 01485 528141
e-mail: info@peacefulpets.co.uk
www.peacefulpets.co.uk

Sympathetic advice and
nationwide cremation service for
horses.

Planning Inspectorate
Zone 4/04
Temple Quay House
2 The Square
Temple Quay
Bristol
BS1 6EB

Appeals to the Secretary of State for
DEFRA.

Prince-Martin and Co
VAT Consultants
Rythorne House
61 Ryland Road
Welton
Lincoln
LN2 3LZ

Pritchard Englefield
Solicitors
14 New Street
London
EC2M 4HE
Tel: 020 7972 9720
e-mail: bgilligan@
  pritchardenglefield.eu.com
www.pritchardenglefield.eu.com

Advice and assistance on most
horse law queries, particularly
horse and rider accident claims.

Redwings Horse Sanctuary
Hall Lane
Frettenham
Nr Norwich
NR12 7RW
Tel: 01603 737432

Horse welfare charity, taking in
rescue cases and some retired
equines.

Riding for the Disabled Association
Avenue R National Agricultural
  Centre
Stoneleigh
Kenilworth
Warwickshire
CV8 2LY
Tel: 024 76 696510

Charity providing riding facilities
for the disabled for pleasure or
rehabilitation.

Royal College of Veterinary
  Surgeons
Belgravia House
62–64 Horseferry Road
London
SW1P 2AF
Tel: 020 7222 2001/08/15
Fax: 020 7222 2004
e-mail: admin@RCVS.org.uk

Professional association and
governing body of veterinary
surgeons, with training and
regulation.

RSPCA
The Causeway
Horsham
West Sussex
RH12 1HG
Tel: 01403 264181
Fax: 01403 241048

Well known welfare charity,
including rescue and rehoming,
and will take on prosecutions for
cruelty to animals.

Society of Master Saddlers (UK)
  Ltd
Kettles Farm
Mickfield
Stowmarket
Suffolk IP14 6BY
Tel: 01449 711642
Fax: 01449 711642

South Essex Insurance Brokers
South Essex House
North Road
South Ockendon
Essex
RM15 5BE
Tel: 01708 859000
Fax: 01708 851520
e-mail: enquiries@seib.co.uk
www.seib.co.uk

Independent brokers offering
advice and provision of equine
insurance needs.

Worshipful Company of Farriers
19 Queen Street
Chipperfield
King's Langley
Herts
WD4 9BT
Tel: 01923 260747
Fax: 01923 261677

Register of farriers, sets
examinations for farriers, and
promotes the welfare of the horse
through raising farriery standards.

Worshipful Company of Saddlers
Saddlers' Hall
40 Gutter Lane
Cheapside
London
EC2V 6BR
Tel: 020 7726 8661/6
Fax: 020 7600 0386

Aims to further the craft of
saddlery and related activities,
including promotion and funding
of training and apprenticeships.

Table of Cases

AC – Law Reports, Appeal Cases
All ER – All England Law Reports
E & B – Ellis and Blackburn
Horse Law – The Equine Law & Litigation Reports (full title). Journal of the Equine Lawyers Association, published bi-monthly
JP – Justice of the Peace & Local Government Review
KB – Law Reports, King's Bench
LT – Law Times Reports
QB – Law Reports, Queen's Bench
RTR – Road Traffic Reports
The Times – the reports in the actual newspaper which may not be reported elsewhere
TLR – Times Law Reports
WLR – Weekly Law Reports

Index